Lymphatic Therapy for Toxic Decongestion

Selected Case Studies for Therapists and Patients

Margaret McCarthy LCSP(Phys) LCSP Register of Remedial Masseurs and Manipulative
Therapists; Remedial Massage Therapist, Reflexologist
Therapist in Private Practice
The North West of England
UK

Foreword by

James L. Oschman PhD
Nature's Own Research Association
Dover
New Hampshire
USA

Illustrations by

Ethan Danioloon

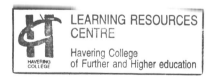
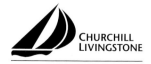
CHURCHILL
LIVINGSTONE

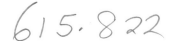

Churchill Livingstone
An imprint of Elsevier Science Limited

First published 2003

ISBN 0 443 07354 6

British Library Cataloguing in Publication Data
A catalogue record for this book is available from the British Library

Library of Congress Cataloging in Publication Data
A catalog record for this book is available from the Library of
Congress

Note
Medical knowledge is constantly changing. As new information
becomes available, changes in treatment, procedures, equipment and
the use of drugs become necessary. The author and the publishers
have taken care to ensure that the information given in this text is
accurate and up to date. However the information given in this text
is for guidance only and is intended only as a supplement not a
substitute for professional tuition and readers are strongly advised to
confirm that the information, especially with regard to vitamin usage
and including all techniques and exercises referred to in this text
comply with the latest legislation and standards of practice. The
author and the publishers accept no liability for any damage, injury
or loss, however caused, which may arise from the information given
in this text (other than as a result of the negligence of the author
and/or the publishers).

The
publisher's
policy is to use
**paper manufactured
from sustainable forests**

Printed in China by RDC Group Limited

Lymphatic Therapy for Toxic Decongestion

For Churchill Livingstone:

Commissioning Editor: Heidi Allen
Project Development Editor: Robert Edwards
Project Manager: Jane Dingwall
Design Direction: George Ajayi

Contents

Foreword

The rapidly growing popularity of complementary therapies has created a vital need for the book you have in your hands. This volume will become a classic, for it breaks new ground in treatment, integrating basic research with clinical practice, and the reporting of new observations. Margaret McCarthy has thoroughly succeeded in her goal of writing for anyone: patient, physician, complementary therapist, or medical researcher. The case studies are fascinating documentaries of real people facing difficult health problems, and struggling to find relief. McCarthy describes her cases with a clear and engaging style, referencing and integrating relevant data from published science. Anatomical terms are thoroughly described and a glossary makes it an easy read for anyone. Her clinical discoveries can help all of us understand ourselves.

In the past, virtually all therapeutic breakthroughs came from laboratories and clinical research centers. Now an important wave of discovery is sweeping through the fields of complementary and alternative medicine. Practitioners of effective, energetic and hands-on therapies are incorporating into their work the best information from modern scientific biomedicine (anatomy, physiology, biochemistry, biophysics, etc). In the process, many persistent and unresolved medical issues are being demystified. This book describes some of these discoveries and makes them readily available for the benefit of both patients and therapists. Eventually basic researchers in fields such as cell and molecular biology should pick up on these important findings and contribute directly to the medicine that is emerging.

While pharmaceutical-based biomedicine continues to make advances, and saves lives on a daily basis, chronic patients are finding their best relief from practitioners of methods that rely more on personal contact, hands-on, and energy methods, or administration of natural substances, often in very low doses. Some of these methods, including those described in this book, teach the patient how to participate in their own healing process, through changes in diet, reducing exposure to toxins in the environment, exercise, and nearly forgotten methods of self massage.

A recurring story is of the suffering patient who has been through batteries of expensive medical tests that have failed to detect any treatable abnormality. Often these patients get the impression that their physicians think they are neurotic or even psychotic. Eventually they may turn to a method that lies outside of conventional medicine, and find a practitioner who gives them a logical and accurate diagnosis, demystifies the symptoms, and begins a successful course of treatment that includes homework. They discover that a whole range of seemingly disconnected symptoms are resolved, once the real source of their problem is pinpointed and treated. Reflection on past conditions all the way back to childhood can reveal patterns that help explain a person's health history. Irritating symptoms such as bloatedness, tiredness, headaches, or obesity may have been signs that the body was being bombarded with chemicals it was not equipped to tolerate and that eventually lead to a health crisis.

McCarthy's treatments focus on the lymphatic system, but other organs and systems are obviously involved. These complex interrelationships are carefully documented in the book.

One important lesson concerns the paradox of the seemingly successful pharmacological intervention. The chronic patient is in pain, and drugs can provide immediate relief. The 'quick fix' may seem to fit with a busy life-style, but it fosters the disastrous illusion that the underlying problem has been resolved. The problem has not been resolved – it has not even been approached. The condition may worsen and the symptoms intensify, leading to an increase in medication, side-effects, and exacerbation of the original problem.

What Margaret McCarthy teaches us about this, is that the drugs and/or their metabolic products, as well as other chemicals in our environment, can accumulate in certain parts of the body. This accumulation process is a natural reaction to the entry of foreign materials that the living system has not experienced before. Rather than allowing these nasty substances to enter the circulation and affect every cell in the body, the organism isolates the materials in lymph nodes, the liver, skin, and other tissues. Eventually accumulations of these strange substances exacerbate a patient's condition, or give rise to other problems that are worse than the original ailment. Other drugs or skin lotions may be prescribed to cope with the side-effects, but these substances must also be dealt with by an already encumbered lymphatic system, creating further imbalance in the body's communication systems. It is important to realize that accumulated poisons probably will not show up in blood or urine tests, because the body has actually taken steps to prevent toxins from reaching these fluids.

Because western medical science has no concept of the vital energetic communication pathways, a confusing and discouraging downward spiral continues. In desperation, an exploratory surgery may be recommended. In other instances, the musculoskeletal system is compromised, structural imbalances arise, and joint replacement is performed. This may bring temporary relief, but the real source of the problem has still not been approached.

We are learning that a physician who recommends joint replacement, without having first tried hands-on or energetic therapies, may be exposing the patient to unnecessary risk, cost, and invasive treatment that can lead to further complications. McCarthy shows how pain medications can settle in a painful region that has poor circulation, leading to problems in nearby joints. The lymphatic system can be encouraged to carry out the functions it is designed for, and the musculoskeletal system can return to its proper structure and function. Joint replacement is a medical miracle, but it should only be utilized when simpler methods have not solved the problem. What is termed 'arthritis' may actually be a symptom of toxic accumulation in the lymphatic system. Similarly, what is called 'asthma' may also be a congestion of the lymphatics.

The approach is appropriately cautious because McCarthy appreciates that the body's filtration systems are delicate and can be damaged if they are suddenly taxed beyond acceptable limits. The protocols seem simple and patients tend to get carried away, but treatments must be tempered by the advice of the therapist because of the possibility of too rapid release and a toxic reaction. This is especially true for the patient who is very ill. And the successful removal of one toxin from the tissues may unmask a deeper layer of accumulation that requires a different approach to neutralization.

Appropriate sequencing and timing of treatments is one of many important contributions McCarthy has made to the therapeutic protocol. And she warns the patient that it is normal if detoxification triggers a temporary worsening of symptoms and even mood swings before improvement begins. Severe headaches and diarrhea are 'the body's way of expressing its eagerness to expel the toxin as quickly as possible and demonstrates just how powerful reflexology can be'.

The careful pace of the therapies, and the recommendation that the patient's condition be followed by their family doctor (in diabetes, for example), results in a powerful and integrated approach to cleansing and strengthening the lymphatic and immune systems. It is an educational approach for both patients and their primary care physicians, who can learn a great deal by watching their patients' steady progress.

There are lessons here for all of us, whether or not we have a chronic ailment: for healthy lymphatic and immune systems may well hold the key to our mutual survival given the rate at which we are adding toxic materials to our environment, and the threats of biological warfare. McCarthy describes exercises that can be practiced daily, while one is in traffic for example, that can keep the lymphatic system tuned-up.

McCarthy also suggests that we look closely at the chemicals in our environment. Dental amalgams used in fillings are extremely toxic, and mercury poisoning affects many people. Some dentists continue to disregard overwhelming evidence on the pathological effects of introducing metals into the mouth. Methods for ridding the body of mercury from fillings are described in Chapter 11. Dental braces can also introduce toxic metals (Chapter 13). These considerations extend to the metals in the items of jewelry that are so popular.

Many people are meticulous about cleanliness, and this is obviously desirable. But over-use of cleaning agents, or any other chemical for that matter, can lead to toxic accumulations in the body and serious health problems. Those who are zealous about cleanliness can profitably direct their attention to the labels on the products they use, and also consider the fumes emitted by appliances such as gas stoves. McCarthy documents how the families of chronically ill patients can become involved in treatment programs by diligently scanning all foods and drinks and cleaning products for toxic ingredients.

McCarthy describes some of the common chemicals, such as the benzoates that are to be avoided, and provides examples of natural, less toxic, and less expensive alternatives to commercial cleaning agents. Lymphatic hygiene begins at home, perhaps under the kitchen sink, where we tend to keep powerful cleansers and other household chemicals. And the discovery of one's food sensitivities can be equally important. There is much valuable information here on nutrition for people with different conditions and sensitivities. Certainly, artificial colors, flavors, and preservatives are to be avoided. Feathers in pillows and various kinds of sprays can also cause problems. Following McCarthy's advice in maintaining a health population of bacteria in the intestines can prevent a wide range of debilitating degenerative disorders before they begin to affect us.

Finally, clinical explorations such as these hold the key to financing our health care system, since it is the chronic and degenerative diseases that consume the largest share of our personal and public resources. The conditions surveyed in this book are common and extremely costly, as they affect a large percentage of the population and prevent many from leading the normal productive quality lives they long for. The lymphatic system holds a major key to public health, yet its possibilities continue to be virtually untapped and ignored. Growing public awareness of the benefits of approaches such as those described here are shifting medicine in a very positive direction.

James L. Oschman 2003

Preface

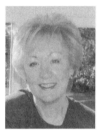

On numerous occasions patients and fellow therapists have asked that I write a book about the integrated therapy I practise. Responding to these wishes, however, left me in a quandary as to which audience I should direct the text – patient or therapist? With some difficulty I have tried to please both.

I wrote this book to heighten the awareness of the lymphatic system and to show its relationship to degenerative disease. I also wanted to demonstrate the hidden power of the lymphatic system, which has been widely overlooked and underutilized. The lymphatic system is the missing link between diagnosis and successful treatment for a wide number of ailments. The intention of this book is to restore normal function to the defense and repair mechanisms within the body – making this principle the primary consideration in any health problem.

Margaret McCarthy 2003

Dedication

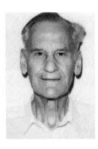

This book is dedicated to Father Fred Fox, a Divine Word missionary priest to whom I owe a great debt of gratitude. Without his unfailing dedication and determination to help his fellow man it would not have been possible to write this book or to help my own family and the many people who have benefited from this therapy. Father Fox's passionate pursuit of knowledge, and his enthusiasm to impart that knowledge unselfishly, inspired me greatly as he encouraged my exploration of complementary medicine, utilizing his research in order to make it available for many people to share as he intended.

And to George, my dear father, who was a dedicated follower of my treatments and their results.

And Catherine, my dear mum, who sadly just missed out on the book's publication.

Margaret McCarthy

Acknowledgments

I'd like to extend my thanks to the following people, without whose help this project would have been impossible.

Without Gary, my son, and his debilitating migraines, I would not have ventured along the road of complementary medicine. His liberation from this condition and his insistence that others be given similar knowledge helped me through the bad days of writing.

My husband, Mike, for his patience and encouragement while writing this book, especially as the manuscript accompanied us on many holidays.

Jeanette, my long-suffering daughter, who talked me through many moments of panic when the computer appeared to devour my work, threatening never to return it. Her support, proofreading and bouquets were invaluable.

Gordon for being so patient during the photographic sessions.

Peggy – for your faith in me.

Andrew Douglas, a dear friend, for his constructive advice.

To my friends – Jim and Molly Vincent, Bette Meek and Sheila King for their valuable input.

To Janice Bray, Louise McVey and Michelle McVey – your contribution to Fred was outstanding, as was your support to me.

To Lydwina for the beautiful hand illustration that is used as Plan 4.

To the many patients and therapists who willed this book along, I extend my sincere appreciation for their belief in the project and for the part they played in the development of my treatment program.

Most of all to my editor, Heidi Allen, who went beyond the call of duty and held my hand when the whole project appeared to be disintegrating. Not forgetting Robert Edwards and his literary mind, whose help with the title was much appreciated.

Introduction

This has not been an easy book to write, due in the main to the teachings of my associate Fred Fox who insisted 'keep it simple'. In keeping it simple I perhaps will not do justice to the pioneers of medicine who, through their findings, laid down the foundations for this therapy. In practice, physical therapists will quickly transcend their teachings and wonder why various parts of the body should present certain disorders. In so doing, the relationship of nerves to muscle groups and various stages of muscle tension resulting in misalignment of bones and restricted blood supply to organs leads to only one conclusion: the body must be viewed as a complete unit. To specialize in the belief that any organic disturbance is of a local nature is a misnomer. We have to remember that circulation of blood and lymph to every cell in the body will not allow for this narrow approach to diagnosis. Fox, in his endeavor to establish a system of assessing the body as a whole, worked towards this objective in his discussions with eminent medical specialists. As a result, in his literature Fox pays tribute to their contribution towards his objective. If in my effort to combine and integrate his teaching and my experience I fail to acknowledge any contribution from others this is not intended, and the fault is entirely mine.

The integrated therapy that is presented as case studies in the second section of the book is a culmination of ancient and new healing techniques. The information criss-crosses between the many functions and systems of the body, as would be expected considering the relationship that exists between symptoms and pathological stages. For this reason I can but touch upon the bare outline of these relationships and the many techniques and therapies that are the basis of this integrated therapy.

Much of the subject matter will, I realize, have been covered by the medically qualified. However, the therapy needs patient participation and for this reason the book has been written from a practical point of view.

To understand the work and research undertaken by Fox, the following quotation from Professor Tiller of Stanford University, California, should prove useful:

Every kind of matter and every organ emits very exact waves. These very weak waves are of an electromagnetic nature and exist in every atom. Every organ has, under normal conditions, its own wave pattern, which distinguishes it from another organ. Harmony among the interplay of wave patterns manifests itself as health; disharmony, as illness. Healing consists in this, that the faulty orientation of the cells in an organ is corrected – brought back into plumb – similar to the way a magnet puts metal shavings into a definite pattern. (Fox, unpublished work, 1988).

The work of Fox was based on what he regarded as the most important discoveries made in the field of biophysics:

1. That the acupuncture points in the body are related energetically to various organs and functions of the body (traditional acupuncture).
2. That the energy levels of the points change with changes in the energy levels of organs and functions (traditional Yang and Yin changes).
3. That the points can be used to energize or sedate organs and functions of the body (traditional acupuncture and moxibustion).
4. That good health ensues when energy balance in the body can be maintained (balance of Yang and Yin).
5. That the traditional Chinese Yang and Yin actually represent the sympathetic and parasympathetic nervous systems.
6. That the energy levels in acupuncture points can be measured electronically by measuring the permeability (electrical resistance) of skin immediately over them with a galvanometer (Kenyon 1983).
7. That the permeability of acupuncture points can be measured even more accurately by removing the skin resistance completely by using more pressure and, if necessary, dampening the skin (Leonhardt 1980).
8. That the chemical or biological causes of energy imbalances in the body can be identified by testing homeopathic antidotes on the body or in the circuit of the measuring device (as recognized by Voll).
9. That the energy levels in the body can be corrected via the acupuncture points using microamp impulses of electricity directly on the points.
10. That energy levels can be corrected in the body by using homeopathic antidotes and remedies (Kenyon 1986).
11. That energy levels can be corrected by using the body's own oscillations which are amplified, inverted or filtered electronically.
12. That energy levels can be corrected by using micromagnetic oscillations, similar to brain waves and the magnetic oscillations of the earth (Hans Brug Institute, see also Oschman 2000).
13. That there are eight additional pairs of meridians in the body apart from the twelve pairs used chiefly in acupuncture (Voll 1982).
14. That the organs and functions of the body are comprehensively represented by more than 250 acupuncture points on the hands and the feet.
15. That there are at least 850 acupuncture points (whose exact relationship to organs and functions has been established by Voll).
16. That the energy levels of individual autonomic nerve plexus and ganglia, as well as of distinct parts of the central nervous system, can be measured on acupuncture points, mainly on the hands, feet, and head (Voll 1982).

Measuring the acupuncture points electronically, it was discovered that disturbance of the energy level of autonomic plexus and ganglia is usually caused by the build-up of toxic substances in lymph nodes adjacent to the plexus and ganglia. The enlarged nodes can be drained and the adjacent nerve ganglia and plexus once cleared of disturbance are then free to innervate the organs and functions of the body adequately (Fox, unpublished work, 1988).

And so it was considered that unless the innervation of organs such as the pancreas, the heart, the glands, the stomach, the duodenum and small intestine, the colon and the lungs can be measured in sufficient detail (individual plexus and ganglia) then deeper causes of many health problems will never be traced. Furthermore, because little or nothing is done to remove the cause of underlying faults within the lymphatic system to allow this innervation to take place it is impossible to give basic treatment.

The discovery by Voll of the eight additional pairs of meridians in the body provides vital information about the nervous system, deep and superficial lymphatics, microcirculation, myelin tissue, connective tissue, skin and joints. It also shows that the acupuncture points in the hands and the feet are a complete system on their own for testing and treating the body; a readily accessible mini-point system. These discoveries make it possible to identify physiological faults in any organ or system of the body quickly and reliably. However, dependence upon instruments for testing has proved to be a major obstacle to their widespread acceptance and use. The protocol for testing devised by Dr Voll also proved to be too complex for most practitioners to master.

Early in 1990, however, Fox discovered that acupuncture points could be tested quickly, easily and objectively simply by touching them with a fingertip and then checking the reaction of the adductor transversus pollicis muscle in the webbing between the thumb and forefinger of the patient's hand. If this muscle thickens, hardens or goes into spasm it is a signal that the information picked up from the acupuncture point by the sensory nerves in the fingertip, and transmitted to the brain, is out of harmony with that person's energy field, and that there is a toxic substance in the vascular or lymphatic system of the organ related to the acupuncture point. If, however, there is no reaction, it means that the related organ is stable. Fingertip testing of acupuncture points opened the way for Dr Voll's discoveries to be made more obtainable to the therapist. This showed the involvement of the lymphatic system in the causation of disorders in the body, and gives us the tools for the harmonizing of energy fields.

There are certain diseases that are so far advanced that nerve reflexes are lost and the nerve impulses so distorted or feeble that it would be impossible to restore normal functioning. In considering treatment, those cases that are amenable to adjustment and the various influences that have bearing upon those changes are described from a very practical viewpoint. Patient participation in the therapy is a requirement for continuity of healing. Therefore, an understanding of the therapies and systems involved in this particular therapy will be discussed from a patient/therapist viewpoint. For the sake of the patient, some detail already known to the therapist is explained further.

REFERENCES

Kenyon J (ed) 1983 Short manual of the VEGATEST method. Bioenergetic regulatory techniques (BER)
Kenyon J 1986 21st century medicine. Thorsons, Northampton
Leonhardt 1980 Fundamentals of electro-acupuncture according to Voll. Medizinisch Literarische Verlagsgesellschaft mbH, Germany
Oschman J 2000 Energy medicine. Churchill Livingstone, Edinburgh, pp 97–100, 183–186
Voll R 1982 Measurement points of the electroacupuncture according to Voll on the hands and feet [transl. H Sarkisyanz]. Medizinisch Literarische Verlagsgesellschaft mbH, Germany

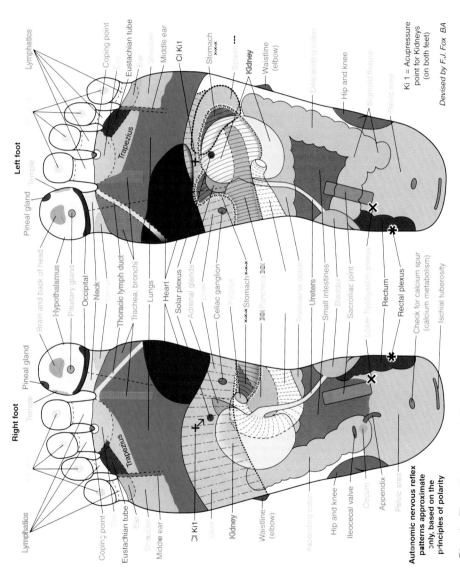

Plan 1 The reflex zones of the foot, plantar view. Organs within the body are at different depths and this is reflected in the reflex chart. Shaded areas on the diagram represent organs that lie deep within the body and the therapist will need to massage through the surface organs first before the deeper ones can be treated. © F. Fox, used with permission.

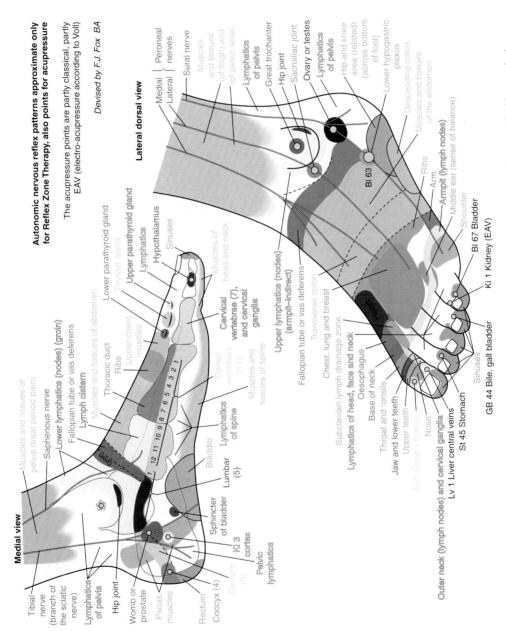

Autonomic nervous reflex patterns approximate only for Reflex Zone Therapy, also points for acupressure

The acupressure points are partly classical, partly EAV (electro-acupressure according to Voll)

Devised by F.J. Fox BA

Lateral dorsal view

Peroneal nerves } Medial / Lateral

Sural nerve

Muscles and tissues (of thigh) and (of pelvic area)

Lymphatics of pelvis

Great trochanter

Hip joint

Sacroiliac joint

Ovary or testes

Lymphatics of pelvis

Hip and knee area (related) (across bottom of foot)

Descending colon

Lower hypogastric plexus

Muscles and tissues of the abdomen

Ribs

Arm

Armpit (lymph nodes)

Middle ear (sense of balance)

Shoulder

Bl 67 Bladder

Ki 1 Kidney (EAV)

Bl 63

GB 44 Bile, gall bladder

Sinuses

St 45 Stomach

Lv 1 Liver central veins

Nose

Sp1 Spleen lymph

Upper teeth

Jaw and lower teeth

Throat and tonsils

Base of neck

Oesophagus

Subclavian lymph drainage zone

Lymphatics of head, face and neck

Outer neck (lymph nodes) and cervical ganglia

Chest, lung and breast

Fallopian tube or vas deferens

Transverse colon

Upper lymphatics (nodes) (armpit–indirect)

Muscles of head and neck

Sinuses

Hypothalamus

Upper parathyroid gland

Lymphatics

Thyroid gland

Lower parathyroid gland

Medial view

Muscles and tissues of abdomen

Upper chest muscles

Ribs

Thoracic duct

Lower lymphatics (nodes) (groin)

Lymph cistern

Fallopian tube or vas deferens

Saphenous nerve

Muscles and tissues of pelvis (treat period pain)

Tibial nerve (branch of the sciatic nerve)

Lymphatics of pelvis

Hip joint

Womb or prostate

Psoas muscles

Rectum

Coccyx (4)

Sacrum (5)

Ki 3 cortex

Pelvic lymphatics

Sphincter of bladder

Bladder

Lumbar (5)

Lymphatics of spine

Muscles and tissues of spine

Dorsal vertebrae (12)

Cervical vertebrae (7), and cervical ganglia

Groin

12 11 10 9 8 7 6 5 4 3 2 1

Plan 2   Reflex zones of the left foot (a) left medial view (b) left lateral and dorsal view. © F. Fox, used with permission.

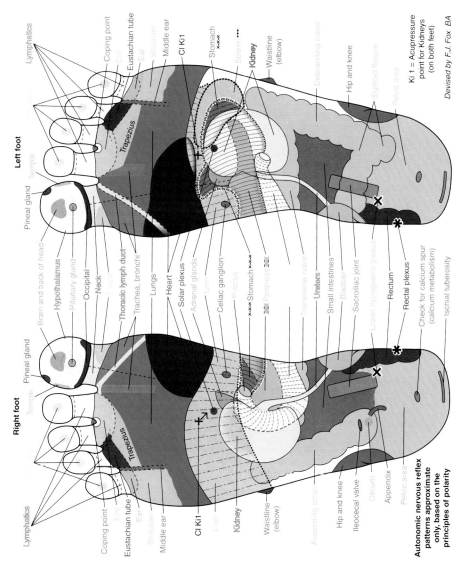

Plan 1   The reflex zones of the foot, plantar view. Organs within the body are at different depths and this is reflected in the reflex chart. Shaded areas on the diagram represent organs that lie deep within the body and the therapist will need to massage through the surface organs first before the deeper ones can be treated. © F. Fox, used with permission.

**Autonomic nervous reflex patterns approximate only
for Reflex Zone Therapy, also points for acupressure**

The acupressure points are partly classical, partly
for Reflex Zone Therapy, also points for acupressure
EAV (electro-acupressure according to Voll)

Devised by F.J. Fox BA

Lateral dorsal view

Sural nerve

Medial ⎱ Peroneal
Lateral ⎰ nerves

Muscles
and tissues
(of thigh) and
(of pelvic area)

**Lymphatics
of pelvis**

Great trochanter

Hip joint

Sacroiliac joint

Ovary or testes

**Lymphatics
of pelvis**

Hip and knee
area (related)
(across bottom
of foot)

Lower hypogastric
plexus

Descending colon

Muscles and tissues
of the abdomen

Ribs

Middle ear (sense of balance)

Shoulder

Arm

Armpit (lymph nodes)

Bl 63

Bl 67 Bladder

Ki 1 Kidney (EAV)

Sinuses

GB 44 Bile, gall bladder

St 45 Stomach

Nose

Sp1 Spleen (lymph)

Upper teeth

Jaw and lower teeth

Throat and tonsils

Base of neck

Oesophagus

Subclavian lymph drainage zone

Lymphatics of head, face and neck

Lv 1 Liver central veins

Outer neck (lymph nodes) and cervical ganglia

Chest, lung and breast

Transverse colon

Fallopian tube or vas deferens

**Upper lymphatics (nodes)
(armpit–indirect)**

Sinuses

Hypothalamus

Lymphatics

Upper parathyroid gland

Thyroid gland

Lower parathyroid gland

Muscles and tissues of abdomen

Ribs

Thoracic duct

Upper chest
muscles

Lower lymphatics (nodes) (groin)

Fallopian tube or vas deferens

Saphenous nerve

Muscles and tissues of
pelvis (treat period pain)

Lymph cistern

Dorsal
vertebrae
(12)

Muscles and
tissues of spine

**Lymphatics
of spine**

Muscles of
head and neck

**Cervical
vertebrae (7),
and cervical
ganglia**

Lumbar
(5)

Bladder

Sphincter
of bladder

Ki 3

Pelvic
cortex

Pelvic
lymphatics

Sacrum
(5)

Coccyx (4)

Rectum

Psoas
muscles

Womb or
prostate

Hip joint

**Lymphatics
of pelvis**

Tibial
nerve
(branch of
the sciatic
nerve)

Medial view

12 11 10 9 8 7 6 5 4 3 2 1

Plan 2 Reflex zones of the left foot (a) left medial view (b) left lateral and dorsal view. © F. Fox, used with permission.

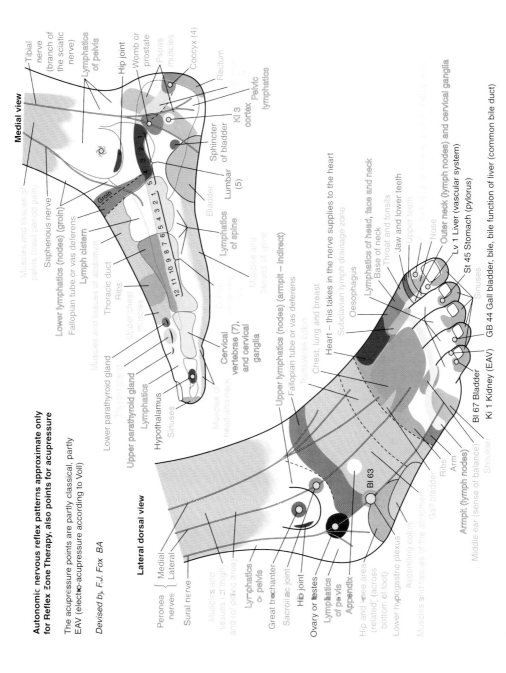

Autonomic nervous reflex patterns approximate only for Reflex Zone Therapy, also points for acupressure

The acupressure points are partly classical, partly EAV (electro-acupressure according to Voll)

Devised by F.J. Fox BA

Medial view

Tibial nerve (branch of the sciatic nerve)
Muscles and tissues of pelvis (real period pain)
Saphenous nerve
Lymphatics of pelvis
Hip joint
Womb or prostate
Psoas muscles
Coccyx (4)
Rectum
Lower lymphatics (nodes) (groin)
Fallopian tube or vas deferens
Lymph cistern
Groin
Lower parathyroid gland
Thyroid gland
Thoracic duct
Ribs
Upper chest muscles
Muscles and tissues of abdomen
Sphincter of bladder
Ki 3 cortex
Pelvic lymphatics
Bladder
Lumbar (5)
Lymphatics of spine
Muscles and tissues of spine
Upper parathyroid gland
Lymphatics
Hypothalamus
Sinuses
Cervical vertebrae (7), and cervical ganglia
Muscles of head and neck

Lateral dorsal view

Peronea nerves { Medial, Lateral
Sural nerve
Muscles and tissues of thigh and (of pelvic area)
Lymphatics of pelvis
Great trochanter
Sacroiliac joint
Hip joint
Ovary or testes
Lymphatics of pelvis
Appendix
Hip and knee area (related) (across bottom of foot)
Lower hypogastric plexus
Muscles and tissues of the abdomen

Upper lymphatics (nodes) (armpit – indirect)
Fallopian tube or vas deferens
Transverse colon
Chest, lung and breast
Heart – this takes in the nerve supplies to the heart
Subclavian lymph drainage zone
Oesophagus
Lymphatics of head, face and neck
Base of neck
Throat and tonsils
Jaw and lower teeth
Upper teeth
Nose
Outer neck (lymph nodes) and cervical ganglia
Lv 1 Liver (vascular system)
St 45 Stomach (pylorus)
Sinuses
GB 44 Gall bladder, bile, bile function of liver (common bile duct)
Ki 1 Kidney (EAV)
Bl 67 Bladder
Arm
Ribs
Gall bladder
Armpit (lymph nodes)
Middle ear (sense of balance)
Shoulder
Ascending colon
Bl 63

Plan 3   Reflex zones of the right foot (a) right medial view (b) right lateral and dorsal view. © F. Fox, used with permission.

Small intestine ●

4 Duodenum, upper horizontal portion
3 Duodenum, descending portion
2 Duodenum, interior horizontal portion
1c Peritoneum
1b CMP small intestine
1a Superior mesenteric plexus
1 Ileum, ileocecal valve

Endocrine system ○

3 Pituitary gland; pineal gland
2 Parathyroid, thyroid and thymus
1d Mammary gland
1c Pancreas: islets of Langerhans
1b CMP
1a Cervical ganglia
1 Adrenals

Circulation ●

7 Coronary vessels
7a Coronary plexus
8 SMP veins   ⎫
8a Right sympathetic trunk   ⎬ Palm side
8b Lymph cistern   ⎭
8c Abdominal aortic plexus
8d CMP
8e Cardiac ganglia
8f Lymph drainage of blood vessels
9 SMP arteries

Colon – large intestine ●

5 MP for proximal wrist joint
4a Appendix and ileocecal lymph nodes
4 Cecum
3a Great omentum
3 Ascending colon
2 Flexure of the colon
1c Peritoneum
1b CMP
1a Superior hypogastric plexus
1.1 Lymph drainage
1 Transverse colon

Lymph drainage ●

5 Lymph drainage of the heart
4b Pharynx and larynx
4a Esophagus
4 Lungs
3 Nose and sinuses
2a Eye
2 Upper and lower jaw
1a Tubal tonsil
1.2 CMP (tonsils)
1.1 Ear
1 Palatine tonsil and cervical lymph nodes

A

Devised by F.J. Fox BA
This illustration from an adaptation by Lydwina Farrell, with permission

Heart ⬤

6   Myocardium
6a Pacemaker
8   Right. Tricuspid valve. Left. Mitral valve
8a Pericardium and subpericardium, lymph vessel network
8b Endocardium
8c CMP for heart
8d Myocardial lymph vessel network
8e Cardiac plexus
8f Subendocardial lymph vessel network
9   Right. Aortic valve. Left. Pulmonary valve

Organs ⬤

1   Abdomen and minor pelvis
1.1 Faulty lymphatics
1a   Faulty ANS
1b   CMP (organs)
1c   Peritoneum
1d   Pleura
2   Chest and neck
3   Head
4   Abdomen/pelvis (alt.)
5   Chest and neck (alt.)
6   Head (alt.)

Allergies ⬤

1   Abdomen, pelvis and legs
1a   Allergic irritation of the A.N.S
1b   C.M.P. Allergy
1c   Vascular sclerosis
2   Skin upper extremities: organs of chest and neck
3   Skin and all organs of the head

Nervous system ⬤

4   C.M.P. for cranial nerves
3a   C.M.P. parasympathetic ganglia/cranium
3   Brain – stem and cerebrum
2   Cervical and thoracic marrow
1c   IC Meninges and spinal marrow
1b   C.M.P. for peripheral and C.N.S.
1a   SMP A.N.S.
1   Lumbar and sacral marrow

Lungs ⬤

9   Trachea
9a   Bronchial plexus
10   Bronchi
10a Pleura
10b Bronchioles
10c C.M.P. for lung
10d Mediastinal plexus
11   Lung parenchym and alveoli

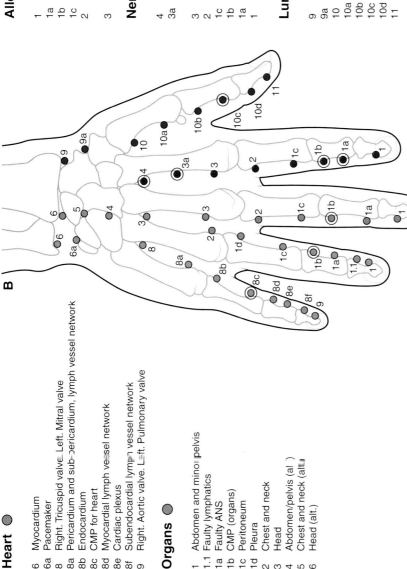

B

Devised by F.J. Fox E4
This illustration from an adaptation by Lydwina Farrell, with permission

Plan 4   Right hand acupuncture points after to Voll 1982. The points illustrated are for fingerpoint testing, assessment, and acupressure only. alt., organs 4, 5 and 6 are alternative points for finger amputees; ANS, autonomic nervous system; CMP, control measurement point; MP, measurement point; SMP, summation measurement point. With thanks to Lydwina Farrell for the beautiful illustration, adapted from the original plan by Father Fox.

Eliminating a narrow approach to diagnosis

The first section of the book gives background information and findings of many eminent bio-physicists. It demonstrates how an integrated therapy drawing on a variety of approaches can assess the body as a whole and in a unique form that promotes healing from within, successfully and without the use of expensive equipment. The response of the immune system to external hazards is the dominant component of this assessment. Congestion within the lymphatic system is proposed as a basis of energy disturbance as elements get trapped in lymph nodes where they build up a magnetic field that is large enough to interfere with nerve signals and ultimately the physiological processes that depend upon those signals. Contraindications to lymphatic drainage will direct the therapist and patient to the filter-clearing procedures prior to any lymphatic movement.

1

Bioenergy in crisis:
the lymphatic connection

There is no single life force or healing energy.
Instead, there are many systems in the body that
conduct various kinds of energy and information
from place to place.　　　　　(Oschman 2000, p 2)

Two systems that circulate the body conveying
this information are the venous and lymphatic
systems. In 1670, Robert Hooke discovered for
the first time what every schoolchild now learns
in elementary biology lessons, that we, and all
creatures on this planet, are created out of incal-
culable individual cells and the fluids that flow
between them. Yet, much of this fluid – that of the
lymphatic system – is usually referred to only in
the presence of cancerous conditions, in the con-
text of the spreading of the disease to adjacent
nodes and channels. This is despite the fact that
any disturbance and organic involvement, from
colds to fevers, will involve the lymphatic system
and that it is, therefore, quite impossible to consider any organic disturbance that does not include
a lymphatic change.[1]

The lymphatic system thus appears to be a
minor consideration in pathology yet is emerging
as the missing link in the cause of physiological
faults that lead to degenerative diseases.

[1] Although old now, F P Millard's *Applied anatomy of the
lymphatics* is nevertheless relevant and well worth
consulting on this subject (see the Reference list). Millard
approaches the topic from the perspective of an osteopath
and his observations remain of great interest.

THE LYMPHATIC SYSTEM AND MICROMAGNETIC POISONING

A toxin or poison is anything that causes injury or death by contaminating a living organism. Such contamination is usually understood to be chemical and its effect is often swift, for example, snake venom or arsenic.

However, there is also a more subtle type of poison, which greatly affects people's health. This is called micromagnetic poison, and it can cause injury, illness and even death, by a gradual breakdown of body tissue and organs.

The health problems that follow micromagnetic poisoning are often classified as psychosomatic in origin – and are said to be caused by the figurative poison of bad attitudes, emotions or memories, for the want of correct diagnosis. One of the most common such problems is stress.

Micromagnetic poisoning is, of course, the end product of contamination by very small magnetic forces or fields that are out of harmony with the body's own magnetic fields.

As we view the lymphatic system in its entirety, as a complete system within itself, and recall its important relationship to almost every tissue and organ, we must realize its significance: the role it plays in its close relationship to tissues in nourishment, secretion and elimination, or purification and infection; the immediate activities of the nodes and channels whether a finger is cut or a throat is infected; the long tinted lines when blood poisoning has started through an infected abrasion; the locating and collection of septic materials that help to prevent sudden poisoning. This is micromagnetic poisoning.

The lymphatic system is constantly charged with infectious material. The vasomotor arrangement in relation to the nodes and ducts and the nerve centers from which impulses come are included in this complex system. The function of the system is to purify or clarify the contents of its nodules, channels and ducts. However, enlarged nodes are often at a distance from the point of infection or tissue poisoning and organic abnormality can cause this system to become blocked and taxed from the points of infection to the termination of the ducts (Millard 1922).

For example, abrasions or insect bites are often given little attention until there is evidence of blood poisoning. This should not be the case, for once the skin has been damaged the lymphatic system will want to deal with the inevitable infection, however insignificant the abrasion. A swelling in the hand as a consequence of an abrasion can result in a tinted or darkened line from the wrist to the axillary nodes in the armpit. When the axillary nodes in the reflex zones of the feet (Fig. 1.1) (the side of the ankle; upper lymphatics indirect) are massaged each day, the swelling in the hand, which could have persisted for 1 month, can disappear within 1 week (Berkson 1977). In this way, patients with autonomic innervation faults diagnosed by electronic or fingertip measurement of acupuncture points receive lymphatic drainage by way of reflexology. Quite remarkably, nerve plexuses previously registering a low energy output now register normal as toxic matter lodged in the lymphatics is removed.

Every element has its own micromagnetic field, built up by electrons as they spin around the nucleus. When molecules of any element, or combination of elements, become trapped in lymph nodes they can build up a micromagnetic

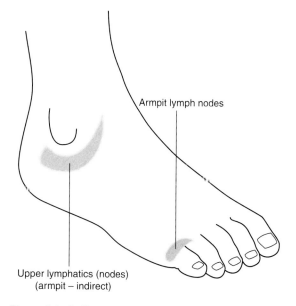

Figure 1.1   Indirect axillary nodes in the reflex zones of the feet.

field that is large enough and strong enough to affect the micromagnetic field generated by nerve signals from the plexus or ganglia. In this way, trapped elements interfere with the nerve signals themselves and, ultimately, with the physiological processes that depend upon those signals (Coghill 1992, p 48).

Correcting any disturbance of nerve signals requires the careful drainage (by lymph drainage exercises) of lymph nodes and tissues in close proximity to any plexus or ganglia. It is interesting to note how toxic matter trapped on one organ can affect physiological processes in a neighboring organ. Substances adhering to the wall of the duodenum can affect the pancreas and result in faulty fat, carbohydrate, protein or nucleoprotein metabolism. Hypoglycemia can develop quite rapidly in this way, the symptoms of which are: anxiety, crying without reason, tremor of the hands and/or body. Remarkably, the most common cause of this phenomenon is rapid detoxification of the body through the lymphatics, blood, spleen, liver and bile system (athletes often display these symptoms after a race). It would appear that much toxic matter stored in fatty tissue is released by exercise, the reaction being due to inappropriate filtering of the toxic matter by the liver, kidneys, spleen and lungs (see Chapter 4).

THE BRAIN AND MICROMAGNETIC POISONING

Although the blood–brain barrier prevents most toxic matter from entering the cerebral fluid, minute particles can get through at times, especially when the blood is severely overloaded due to inadequate filtration of the filters (i.e. the liver, kidneys, spleen or lungs). Such congestion of toxic matter acts as a focus on the brain. This focus can usually be traced by measuring the acupuncture points related to different parts of the brain and their causes identified by testing with micromagnetic antidotes (Ludwig 1983). The toxins, which are thought to adhere in the capillary beds, can be cleared from this area by various techniques. This often requires great patience and persistence, as the focus might be very deep-seated in the brain and become

apparent on the acupuncture points only as the toxins begin to break loose and become trapped in related areas (Walton 1981, p 1291) (see Chapter 15). The focus can keep recurring until the toxins have been filtered out of the blood by the filters. Unless these filters are functioning to their optimum efficiency, lymphatic drainage will not be effective and toxic matter will pollute the cerebral fluid, eventually ending up in some other part of the brain.

Most commonly, toxic matter becomes trapped and forms a focus in the network of capillaries themselves, which make up the choroid plexus or which supply tissue fluid (i.e. interstitial fluid; Smith 1990, p 996) to the pituitary gland and the hypothalamus. One of the most vulnerable areas is the lateral ventricle on the right side of the brain. The temporal horn of the ventricle (behind the temple) lies adjacent to the hippocampus and amygdala, two parts of the limbic system. The former controls the formation of new memories and the sleep–waking cycle; the latter controls emotions such as fear, anger and sexual attraction. Sedation of the amygdala can cause docility and lack of emotional response; stimulation can cause inappropriate fear, claustrophobia, agoraphobia, anger and aggressive behavior. Other very vulnerable parts of the brain are the brainstem and, closely associated with it, the pineal gland (Barr & Kiernan 1983, pp 264–271) (further details in Chapter 15).

THE INTESTINAL TRACT AND MICROMAGNETIC POISONING

A further example of micromagnetic poisoning takes place in the intestinal tract and affects the enteric nervous system. This system consists of nerve cells within the wall of the intestine; these nerve cells stimulate peristalsis. Peristalsis not only brings about the mixture and movement of intestinal contents (chyme, fiber and wastes) but also ensures efficient absorption of nutrients. When something adheres to the intestinal wall, the enteric nervous system is weakened or cancelled in that area. It would appear that the otherwise harmless fungus *Candida albicans* can take root on the wall of the intestine, dampen the enteric system even more and eventually release spores into the bloodstream, which can in turn cause agglutination and foci in the circulatory system. *Candida* in the bloodstream is perceived by the body as 'foreign' and can therefore evoke an immune reaction. A number of personality problems ranging from depression, sudden mood swings and even schizophrenic symptoms can be the result of these spores reaching the brain (Berg 1983).

CONCLUSION

Micromagnetic poisoning is a major factor in diseases of many kinds. As Kenyon observes, there is a consensus, which includes the medical profession, that treating the cause is the best way of coping with any illness (Kenyon 1986, p 29). Finding the cause through information provided via acupuncture points, eliminating toxins through lymphatic drainage techniques, reflexology and finally via the filters is a most significant approach in the treatment of ill-health and disease today.

REFERENCES

Barr M L, Kiernan J A 1983 The human nervous system. Harper & Row, New York

Berg R 1983 Human intestinal microflora in health and disease. Academic Press, London

Berkson D 1977 The foot book. Harper & Row, New York

Coghill R 1992 Electrohealing. Thorsons, London

Kenyon J N 1986 21st century medicine. Thorsons, Northampton

Ludwig W 1983 Fundamental principles of Mora therapy. Hans Brugemann-Institute, Germany

Millard F P 1922 Applied anatomy of the lymphatics. Australia: International Lymphatic Research Society. (Available from: Health Research, PO Box 850, Pomeroy, Western Australia 99347)

Oschman J 2000 Energy medicine. Churchill Livingstone, Edinburgh

Smith A (ed) 1990 The British Medical Association Complete Family Health Encyclopedia. Dorling Kindersley, London, p 996

Walton 1981 Neurology. In: Smith L H, Thier S O (eds) Pathophysiology: The Biological Principles of Disease (International Textbook of Medicine, Vol. 1). W B Saunders, Philadelphia, p 1291

FURTHER READING

Draser B S, Hill K J 1974 Human intestinal flora. Academic Press, London

Jayasuriya A Clinical acupuncture. Sri Lanka: The Acupuncture Foundation

Kurz I 1996 Textbook of Dr Vodder's manual lymph drainage, vol. 3, 3rd edn. Karl F Haug Verlag GmbH & Co, Belgium

Oldfield H, Coghill R 1998 The dark side of the brain. Elements Books, Dorset

2

Uncovering the body's hidden language and the discovery of the immune system response

There is little doubt that the immune system responds physiologically to external hazards, yet few of us take advantage of the mechanisms and protective capabilities this system provides. The efficiency of the immune system is dependent upon a competent lymphatic system, the protection of which will be limited if it is constantly being furnished by external hazards. What is not appreciated is the body's highly organized defense and repair equipment, which must be utilized if there is to be any advance in the fight against degenerative disease. This chapter will introduce the tools by which any external hazard can be identified and eradicated.

The webbing of the right hand that forms between the thumb and forefinger has become a significant asset in the simplified version of a complex therapy. An interesting relationship was established between a muscle spasm in this adductor transversus pollicis (ATP) muscle and tension in the area around the base of the neck. The ATP muscle is the only muscle of the hand, that shares its sympathetic nerve supply with the thymus in the chest. The thymus is a central organ of the immune system whose nerve supply comes from the thoracic ganglia T2. Whenever any toxic substance, false idea or bad emotion stresses the immune system the muscles react to the stress by a distinct thickening or spasm. This is known as an immune system response (ISR) and this response is felt in the ATP muscle in the

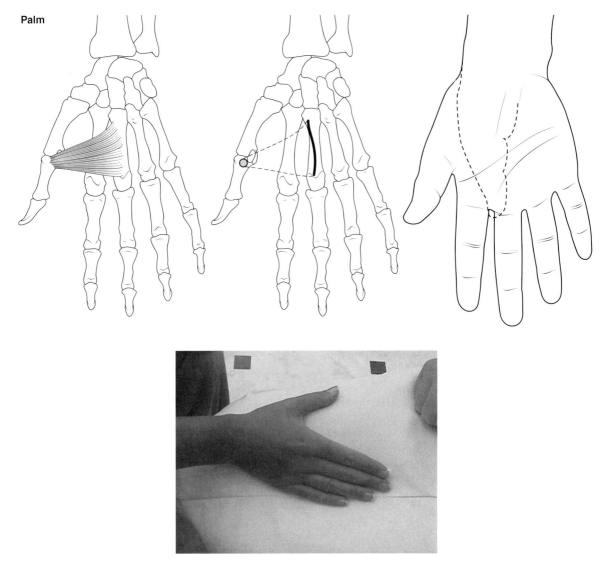

Figure 2.1 The adductor transversus pollicis muscle.

webbing of the hand (Fig. 2.1). This will be discussed further, on p 11.

REFLEXOLOGY

The benefits of reflexology, along with its application, are instrumental in the improvement of those people who are featured in the case studies in section two of this book. For this reason, a significant account of the therapy, together with informative charts, is provided in an easy-to-follow format relative to each case study (see Chapter 5).

ELECTRO-ACUPOINT TESTING

Dr Reinhold Voll was among the first to realize that the electromagnetic emissions from the body and brain offered the possibility of diagnosis. Voll found that electrical resistance was considerably different when patients were ill than when they were healthy, and discovered that the acupuncture point was electrically negative with respect to its surrounding skin. He built a complicated system of disease diagnosis based on this discovery and was involved in the development of the Vegatest machine. Using this machine, with the flow of energy through the acupuncture points Voll discovered the exact relationship of hundreds of acupuncture points to specific parts of the body and functions within the body. He detected that the acupuncture points on the fingers and toes, as well as the hands and feet, contain vital information about all the organs and systems of the body (Voll 1978).

Since its birth in 1953, electro-acupoint testing (otherwise known as electro-acupuncture according to Voll (EAV)) has developed into an extensive method for testing the body in great detail. This is achieved by determining the correct energy flow that passes through the acupuncture points. Voll found that, in disease, the voltage indicator fell, but could be corrected by determining which homeopathic remedies, herbs or drugs were most suitable to renew the energy to that point. Having found out which remedies arrested falls in the indicator, Voll applied these to the patient with good results. However, the Vegatest approach depended on a high level of operator skill to find which substance would actually balance the circuit and therefore treat the patient. Although Voll's concepts were adopted in Germany, they did not find much favor elsewhere because of the reliance on the skill of the operator to apply the correct pressure to the acupuncture point (Coghill 1992, p 39).

Franz Morrell, a colleague of Voll, further discovered how to administer the precise homeopathic treatment simply and effectively using EAV. Together with his son-in-law, E. Rasche, an electronics expert, Morrell invented the Mora machine (a combination of the first two letters from each name), a very sophisticated electronic instrument that could apply the correct potency of homeopathic remedy directly to the body. This was achieved using information taken directly from the patient's body as he or she held an electrode that was attached to the Mora machine. This information was used to identify a homeopathic remedy

and the correct potency was administered via the acupuncture points using an electrode (Fox, personal communication, 1986).

HOMEOPATHY

To understand how homeopathy works one must realize that everything radiates magnetic energy: Every chemical and microbe, every mineral, plant and living being radiates a magnetic field that is unique.

Homeopathic remedies are prescribed under what the Society of Homeopaths calls the Law of Similars. This law states that 'what makes you sick shall heal'. The society believes that the symptoms that are caused by an overdose of a substance are the symptoms that can also be cured by a very small dose of the same substance. The remedies, which are derived from plants, minerals, metals or poisons, are prepared by dilution and violent shaking in a solution of alcohol and water. This process is described as potentization and is done from three or four to many thousands of times. Frequently, the dilution is so great that no chemical trace of the original substance remains, and these high dilutions are regarded by homeopaths as their most potent remedies. There is abundant proof that homeopathic remedies *do* work, but scientists have yet to agree on *how* they work. They believe that the answer is to be found in the field of electromagnetism. The process of dilution and violent shaking, it is claimed, apparently imprints the characteristic energy pattern of the original substance on the liquid in which it is diluted. A homeopathic remedy acts as a signal, that energizes or stimulates the body's self-healing powers (Fletcher 1993, p 207).

Electromagnetic fields are characterized by the phenomenon of vibration and everything exists in a state of vibration or frequency, which can be measured. The entire mechanisms of vibrational or energy medicine were explored in 1988 by the physician Richard Gerber. Gerber suggests that human organisms are a series of interacting multidimensional subtle energy systems and that if these systems become unbalanced there will be resulting pathological symptoms. However, he describes how rebalancing the subtle energy with vibrational medicine can heal these imbalances (Coghill 1992, pp 109–110). For example, a homeopathic remedy works in the following way: When two opposing magnetic fields are applied simultaneously to the body they cancel-out or neutralize each other's energy fields. Provided, of course, that the correct remedy can be identified. An example of this counteraction of magnetic fields is described in Chapter 3.

ACUPUNCTURE POINTS

Acupuncture started in China several thousand years ago. The Chinese consider that energy circulates in the body along specific channels, which they call meridians. This flow of energy has a direction and the Chinese decided that the balance of energy from side to side, top to bottom and from the inside to the outside of the body was of great importance. They expressed this idea using the principle of Yin and Yang, which considers that everything is an amalgam of opposites (the opposites being called Yin and Yang). Yang was associated with activity, fire and light (or the male principle) and Yin was associated with physical substance and water (or the female principle). The balance between these two opposites was considered to be a vigorous balance. If a person was out of balance in an energetic sense then the principle of treatment would be to re-establish that balance. The Chinese believed that, as well as being in balance, the energy or life force (chi) had to be able to circulate freely around the meridians. If there was a break in its circulation anywhere then illness would result (Bai Xinghua & Baron 2001).

It is precisely this definition of freely circulating energy that is applied when using EAV testing. By reading the energy that is flowing through these acupuncture points, which are located along energy lines called meridians, an imbalance can be identified.

We must acknowledge the great strides that Dr Voll and his colleagues made in developing this technology and gaining the attention of many eminent people who were prepared to take his research further.

ADDUCTOR TRANSVERSUS POLLICIS

After much searching and testing using EAV, and after healthy discussion and transfer of information between therapists, it was eventually discovered that the ATP muscle will always form a spasm in the hand when pressure is exerted on one of the upper thoracic vertebrae. It was eventually established that the spasm in the webbing of the hand always forms when a muscle spasm forms over the spine in the area of the second thoracic vertebra, and that this happens whenever the thymus is stressed. What was in fact discovered was that the acupuncture point B1 12 in the spinal area is the associated (Yu) point for the thymus. It became clear that whenever the thymus (which comprises central immune tissue) is stressed, a muscle spasm forms over one or both sides of the second thoracic vertebra, depending upon whether only one side or both sides of the thymus are involved. The ATP muscle spasm in the webbing of either hand forms whenever the second thoracic spinal nerve on the corresponding side of the body is compressed by a muscle spasm forming over it. Remarkably, the ATP muscle spasm forms in the webbing of the right hand whenever any toxic matter adheres to immune tissue (papillia vaeri) at the end of the common bile duct on the wall of the duodenum. It also forms in the webbing of the left hand whenever toxic matter attaches to the immune tissue (Peyer's patches) on the wall of the jejunum. Most remarkably, the ATP muscle spasm forms in the webbing of both hands whenever any substance out of harmony with the immune system or the digestive system, the pancreas (indirectly through lack of secreted enzymes entering the duodenum) is placed in either hand, touched with any fingertip, placed most anywhere on the body or put within range of the biomagnetic field of the body (within a centimeter or two of the skin).

The advantage of these phenomena is twofold. First, toxic matter can be identified by having the patient touch or hold in the hand various antidotes: for chemical or disease. As soon as the correct antidote or combination of antidotes is in contact with the body, the immune system will cease to be stressed and the ATP muscle spasm will immediately disappear. Alternatively, toxic matter can be identified by placing the super snooper (see Chapter 13) over suspected substances on the body, i.e. ornaments, make-up, shampoo, antiperspirant, soap powder, dental fillings. As soon as the magnetic flux encounters a toxin it neutralizes the toxin magnetically ('homeopathically') and the spasm in the hand disappears.

Second, simply having the patient touch the remedies can identify an appropriate homeopathic remedy. If the appropriate remedy is related to a comparatively recent health problem it will most likely act mainly in support as a drainage remedy, helping the body to expel toxic matter from organs, connective tissue and even joints. If the remedy is related to deep-seated toxins, such as an inherited factor (for example, tuberculinum) the remedy will most likely be constitutional and should help the patient mentally and emotionally as well as physically (Fox, unpublished work, 1990).

Birthmarks

Birthmarks usually contain traces of inherited factors and so can be very useful in determining constitutional remedies. Simply have the patient touch a birthmark with a finger and then test which remedy is appropriate, as described above (Fox, unpublished work, 1990).

This discovery was aptly named immune system response (ISR). The ISR can be used in clinical situations where an electrode cannot be used, for example, on a child suffering from eczema, where the broken skin would distort the information. The implications of these discoveries are immense because they open up the possibility for bioenergetic testing objectively and without dependence upon instruments or operator competency. This allows for the energy state of any organ to be assessed and, if necessary, the appropriate medication or homeopathic remedy given to prevent the progress of disease.

REFERENCES

Bai Xinghua M D, Baron R B 2001 Acupuncture visible holism. Butterworth-Heinemann, Oxford
Coghill R 1992 Electrohealing. Thorsons, London
Fletcher E 1993 The optimum health guide. Hodder & Stoughton, London
Voll R 1978 Organs, fields of disturbance, and tissue systems [transl. H Schuldt]. Medicina Biologica, Germany

FURTHER READING

Adams P 1997 Natural medicine for the whole person. Element Books, Dorset
Castro M 1991 The complete homeopathy handbook. Macmillan, London
Jing Chen 1982 Anatomical atlas of Chinese acupuncture points. Shandong Science and Technology Press, Jinan, China
Kenyon J 1987 Acupressure techniques. Thorsons, Northampton
Lockie A, Geddes N 1995 The complete guide to homeopathy – the principles of practice and treatment. Dorling Kindessley, London
Voll R, Sarkisyanz H 1983 The 850 EAV measurement points of the meridians and vessels including secondary vessels [transl. A J Scott-Morley]. Medicina Biologica, Germany

USEFUL ADDRESS

The Society of Homeopaths
2 Artizan Road, Northampton, NN1 4HU
Tel: 01604 621400

3

How to use the immune system response

Professor Jonathon Brostoff, Consultant to the Allergy Clinic, The Middlesex Hospital, London, recommends an environmental approach to diseases. He emphasizes that both environmental factors and foods play a significant part in chronic ill health today and stresses that if the cause of the disease can be identified and removed, this must be better than suppression of the symptoms by drugs. This approach to disease uses information from cost–benefit analyses to show considerable savings in healthcare costs to the Exchequer and, above all, considerable benefit to the overall health of the individual (Action Against Allergy 1998).

The adductor transversus pollicis (ATP) muscle can assist in this environmental approach and in the identification of substances that could cause an adverse reaction to the body (see Chapter 2). The test is easy to use and relays a lot of information to the therapist on the suitability of food and any other substance for the patient. Furthermore, acupuncture points can quickly, easily and objectively be tested using this method.

THE HOMEOPATHIC AND ACUPUNCTURE CONNECTION

Most toxic substances are well buffered in body tissue and do not always register on acupuncture points. In the course of lymphatic drainage they emerge one after the other (identified through EAV and fingertip testing) into the vascular system, where they affect the autonomic innervation. Then the acupuncture points related to the affected areas react and register disharmony. If a health problem is related to any organ, that organ must be tested and treated repeatedly in the course of therapy. The muscle reaction in the webbing of the hand is related to a reaction of the thalamus and thymus to sensory information. The thalamus is in direct receipt of the information and relays its reaction to the thymus. If the information causes stress, the reaction immediately affects the ATP muscle because it shares its sympathetic innervation (the second thoracic ganglion on the spine) with the thymus. Because the thymus is central immune tissue, the reaction in the muscle indicates an immune system response (ISR).

The moment a disharmonic acupuncture point on the body is touched, or an allergen comes into bodily contact, a spasm forms immediately in the ATP muscle.

Fingertip testing of acupuncture points opens the way for identifying physiological faults throughout the body:

1. In the immune system: bone marrow, thymus, spleen and lymph nodes.
2. In the nervous system: central and peripheral; sympathetic and parasympathetic; sensory and motor; also the enteric nervous system.
3. In the endocrine system: each gland has at least two points.
4. In the circulatory system: heart, arteries, veins, vascular system, lymphatic system. The heart alone has 36 points in the hands.
5. In the respiratory system: lungs, bronchi, pleura and trachea.
6. In the digestive system: stomach, small intestine and pancreas.
7. In the excretory system: colon, kidneys and bladder.
8. In the structural system: joints, connective tissue and fatty tissue.
9. In the reproductive system: penis, seminal vesicles, ovarian duct, womb, etc.

Furthermore, the additional eight pairs of meridians discovered by Voll offer a readily accessible mini-point system that is ideal for fingertip testing and therapy (Fox, unpublished work, 1992).

Although it is possible to feel the spasm in the webbing of both hands, the right hand will be used in all of the following tests (Fig. 3.1). The spasm that is felt forming in the adductor muscle is the muscle shortening and thickening. It feels turgid to the touch, like a solid mass or swelling. In its normal, relaxed state, the muscle should feel flaccid. Before trying this technique it must be stressed that this is not a substitute for conventional medicine, although the appropriateness of a drug can be assessed using this technique.

It is very important to practise this technique until you are sure that you can feel the spasm forming. A little massage to the muscle prior to testing is helpful. As this technique is difficult to perform on oneself, you might want to use a surrogate to test yourself (see p 15).

As the spasm forms in the ATP muscle whenever the thymus is stressed, it is worth bearing in mind that the thymus is not able to distinguish between physical, emotional or mental stress. However, this can be a good opportunity to assist a patient whose symptoms stem from an emotional problem. The spasm can be used for identifying a Bach Flower or homeopathic remedy (see Chapter 9).

To clear a spasm in the webbing of the hand before testing

As the spasm in the webbing of the hand is in complete harmony with the duodenum, it

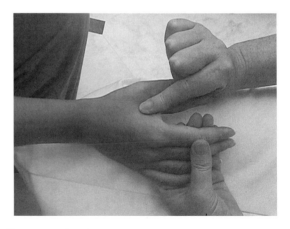

Figure 3.1   Testing the adductor transversus pollicis muscle for spasm.

follows that if the hand is in spasm the duodenum must be too. Consequently, any spasm that has formed in the duodenum prior to testing must be cleared.

With the patient in a seated position, use the thenar eminence of the right hand to massage quite firmly from just below the ribs on the right side towards the navel (Fig. 3.2); continue until the spasm has subsided. The result will be felt in the webbing of the right hand, from the hard mass of swollen muscle before clearing, to its flaccid state after clearing. The spasm can often feel uncomfortable for the patient. If this exercise has not cleared the spasm tap the patient gently with a clenched fist over the thymus (upper sternum).

It is possible to check the capability of the ATP muscle prior to testing by asking the patient to press a finger against the thymus and hold it there while you feel for the muscle reaction. You should feel a distinct hardening of the muscle. Then ask the patient to remove the pressure and you should detect a distinct softening of the muscle. Repeat the testing until you are familiar with the reaction. The ATP muscle will also react (spasm) if the patient or therapist places the tip of the index finger against an acupuncture point that is out of balance because the part of the body related to that point has an imbalance in the sympathetic and parasympathetic nerve supply. This method can be used to identify health problems, the areas involved and the remedies that are appropriate for therapy.

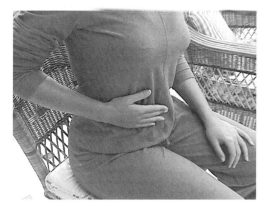

Figure 3.2 Clearing the duodenum prior to testing.

The homeopathic connection

The most crucial task facing a homeopathic practitioner is that of identifying an appropriate remedy for each patient. The conventional method for doing this is reportorization. This method of prescribing can be very time-consuming and complicated, because it entails matching symptoms with remedies that produce and relieve the same health problems. The use of computers programmed for this purpose speeds up the process and limits the choice of remedies to three or five. But the final choice can still be very tricky (Kenyon 1986, p 59). However, using ISR and simply having the patient touch the remedies can identify an appropriate homeopathic remedy.

HOW TO TEST

Hold the right hand of the person to be tested with the palm face down in your left hand. Place the forefinger of your right hand on top of the webbing of the hand while your thumb is underneath, and squeeze the muscle gently between the thumb and forefinger, making sure that the muscle is flaccid (see Fig. 3.1).

To test for substances that are inappropriate for the body

Ask the patient to hold the substance that is being tested for its suitability in the left hand. If a spasm forms in the muscle, then the body will not tolerate that substance.

It is possible to check all foodstuffs in this way, as well as plants, clothes, cosmetics and furniture. Glass vials can be used for the testing of foodstuffs, as glass does not appear to alter the energy field of the substance that is being tested. If a patient is unwell with a cold or flu, and a spasm has formed, do not clear the spasm by massage. Instead, identify a homeopathic remedy to correct the fault, using exactly the same technique. Ask the patient to hold each homeopathic remedy in the left hand while you test the muscle (Fig. 3.3). When the muscle becomes flaccid, the remedy being held is the remedy that will

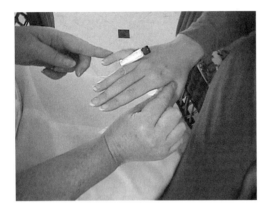

Figure 3.3   Identifying a homeopathic remedy.

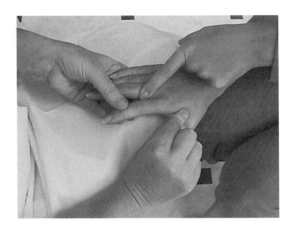

Figure 3.4   Identifying a malfunctioning acupuncture point (lymph cistern).

suit the patient's body at that moment. All the homeopathic remedies that are referred to are at 6c or 30c potency. Homeopathic remedies can be used quite safely in low potencies, if a remedy does not suit a person its energies will go unabsorbed, like radio waves in a radio not tuned into a particular station.

This technique is not intended as a cure-all solution and a medical doctor must be consulted if symptoms persist.

Practice makes perfect!

Practising the technique below on different patients enables the therapist to become familiar with the change in the webbing of the hand. This can be demonstrated repeatedly during the learning process. For example, a substance rich in sulfur (e.g. antidandruff shampoo) will immediately affect the nervous system of the patient. Sensory nerves in the hand pick up the radiation of the sulfur and transmit it to the brain, where the thalamus relays it to the immune system. Then the thymus, which is a central organ of the immune system, reacts and is stressed by the sulfur. This is transmitted to the 2nd thoracic sympathetic ganglion (T2) and from there to the lymphoid tissue at the entrance to the duodenum and to the ATP muscle in the hand, where it causes a spasm. The spasm can be clearly felt in most people. Removal of the substance containing the sulfur from the hand causes the spasm to resolve itself; replacing it causes the spasm to return.

Homeopathic test

However, if the homeopathic remedy Sulfur is taken into the hand together with the sulfur-rich substance, no spasm occurs. This is due to the Sulfur radiating an energy field that cancels out the energy field produced by the sulfur-rich substance. In other words, the homeopathic Sulfur radiates the mirror image energy field to that of the sulfur-rich substance and thereby neutralizes it.

The acupuncture connection

The ATP muscle reaction to fingertip testing of acupuncture points is related to a reaction of the thalamus and thymus. The thalamus is in direct receipt of sensory information and relays its reaction to the thymus. If the information picked up by the fingertip causes stress, the reaction immediately affects the adductor muscle and disharmony in an acupuncture point can be tested in this way with equal success.

The acupuncture points, which are energetically linked with inner organs and parts of the body, can be used to test for any malfunction in the physiological state of the body by touching the point with a fingertip (Fig. 3.4) and then checking the reaction of the muscle. If the ATP thickens, hardens or goes into spasm it is a signal that the information picked up from the point by the sensory nerves in the fingertip and transmitted to the brain is out of harmony with that person's energy field and that there is a toxic substance in the vascular or lymphatic system of the organ related to the point. What this amounts to is that there is now a comparatively simple method for making numerous tests via an immune system response, thus making Dr Voll's discoveries more accessible. On its website (www.eavnet.com), the International Medical Association for EAV states that:

> Modern biophysical research could confirm that higher organisms react to individual electromagnetic signals and that they enter into resonance with particular frequencies. Recent research showed that the process of propagation of the signals takes place in close conjunction with the Chinese Acupuncture meridians. In Germany for example it was Dr Muecke who showed this by experiments with Deuterium that propagated along the meridians and vessels after subcutaneous injection. Furthermore it could be shown that accumulated toxins that are stored in the tissues can interrupt these paths which evokes the so-called blockades. Investigations about different homeopathic substances in different dilutions showed moreover that they are able to emit photons and electromagnetic fields in a very specific pattern.

HOW TO IDENTIFY THE CORRECT HOMEOPATHIC REMEDY

Once a disturbed acupuncture point has been established and the reason identified, a homeopathic remedy might be required to neutralize the disturbed field and to assist the body in the healing process. This is identified by the patient holding each individual remedy in the hand. When the ATP muscle returns to its flaccid state this indicates that the patient's magnetic field has been harmonized and that remedy or combination of remedies is the correct remedy for that patient.

EXCEPTIONS TO THE IMMUNE SYSTEM RESPONSE

There are exceptions for some people who cannot be tested directly. Those with short, thick webbing are difficult to assess, as are others with a defect in

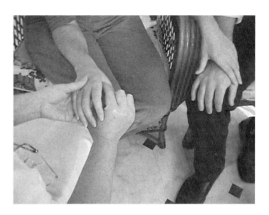

Figure 3.5   Using a surrogate.

the central nervous system, such as motor neuron disease. Those people whose immune system has been suppressed by antibiotics, drugs or disease also do not form a spasm in the hand. It has also been noticed that many people with amalgams or other metals in the mouth register a spasm in the hand at all times (see Chapter 11).

Using a surrogate

It is possible to test babies, the very young and those people mentioned above with a defect in the central nervous system, with the help of a surrogate.

The surrogate's right hand must be spasm free before any testing can commence (to clear the spasm before testing, see pp 12–13) and he or she should place the left hand on the skin of the person to be tested (Fig. 3.5). If a spasm forms immediately then the person being tested already has a spasm in the duodenum. This will also need to be cleared before testing can commence. You can then proceed with the identification of physiological disturbances or the identification of substances that are toxic to the body.

REFERENCES

Action Against Allergy 1998 AAA Newsletter, vol. 62
Kenyon J 1986 21st century medicine. Thorsons, Northampton

FURTHER READING

Werner F, Voll R 1979 Electro-acupuncture primer [transl. H Schuldt]. Medizinisch Literarische Verlagsgesellschaft mbH, Germany

USEFUL ADDRESSES AND CONTACTS

A test kit of homeopathic remedies can be purchased from: Bio-Medscan

Back Sload, Balkram Edge, Wainstalls, Halifax, West Yorkshire HX2 0UB
Tel: 01422 49399
E-mail: stan.richardson@messages.co.uk

More information on acupuncture is available online at: http://www.medical-acupuncture.co.uk/patients.shtml

4

Why are the filters of the body so important?

A COMPROMISED NERVOUS SYSTEM

Whenever massage is used to assist lymphatic drainage, the acupuncture points relating to the massaged area and organs of the body return to their normal energy reading. It is impossible for any of the organic functions of the body to be separated from the result of massage, which causes improved circulation of blood and lymph. The improved circulation relieves the tissues of congestion and bathes them in nutrition through the lymph (see Chapter 5).

THE EFFECTS OF EXERCISE

Exercise increases the frequency of the pulse rate and the quickened blood current during exertion is the result of muscular contraction. Frequent muscular movements cause increased activity in the venous, arterial and lymphatic system, which is essential for health. Exercise, therefore, assists lymphatic drainage and can be instrumental in relieving congestion in the tissues. This is necessary for health, but only if the filters of the body are adequately prepared to receive the sudden influx of toxins the exercise encourages.

FILTERING TOXIC WASTE

Acupuncture points for the liver, kidneys, spleen or lungs (filters) display a distinct reduction in

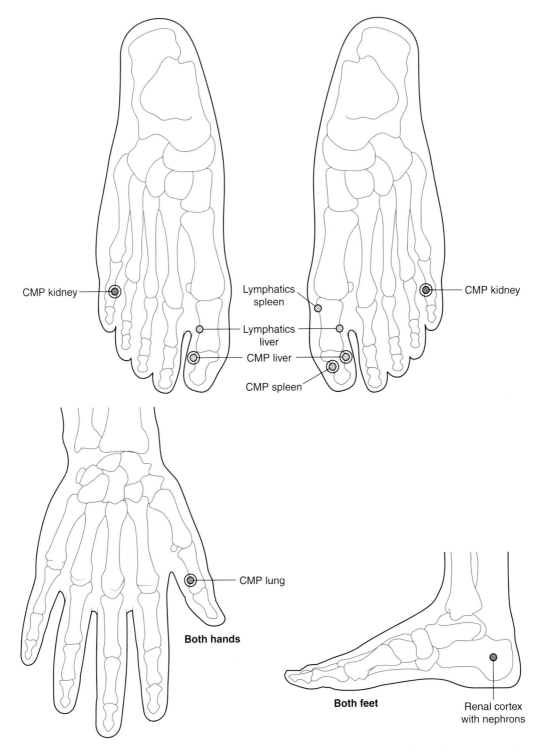

Figure 4.1 Acupuncture points for the filters. The points illustrated are for fingertip testing, assessment, and acupressure only. CMP, control measurement point.

electrical output following any massage. This is due to toxic waste being filtered out of the body through these organs after the massage. The filters will show an altered electrical output after a simple neck and shoulder massage and the substances responsible can be identified through EAV and fingertip testing of the corresponding acupuncture points (Fig. 4.1).

Before lymphatic drainage is encouraged it is therefore advisable to ensure that these filters are functioning to the best of their ability and are not already overwhelmed by any substance that is in the process of being filtered at that time. Headaches are often a sign that the filters are having difficulty processing excess amounts of toxic substances, and a dull ache over the right eye usually signifies that the liver in particular is under pressure.

Processing the body's waste is a very demanding job and the lymphatic system puts pressure on all the filters to do this work efficiently. If the filters are congested before lymphatic drainage commences, they will not be able to effectively remove more waste. As the body does not have an alternative outlet, the toxins will be reabsorbed.

The journey the lymph has to take during lymphatic drainage is complicated and, if laden with toxic waste, unsafe. For the benefit of the patient reading this book this system is explained further.

As the lymph moves through the vessels, collecting toxins as it passes through the complicated system of ducts and lymph nodes, it slowly makes its way to the bloodstream. As it passes through the nodes, the lymph from the majority of the lymphatic vessels collects in the lymph cistern before discharging the contents into its two drainage points (the left thoracic duct and the right lymphatic duct) then finally into the bloodstream.

The lymph cistern

The lymph cistern is a collecting vessel about the size of the little finger; it sits deep in the abdomen. It drains lymph from the lungs, the abdomen and legs before the lymph moves up through the left thoracic duct and into the subclavian vein behind the left clavicle, where it then empties into the bloodstream. The remainder of the lymph from the rest of the body empties into a smaller duct, the right lymphatic duct, which empties into the bloodstream via the subclavian vein, behind the right clavicle at the base of the neck (Fig. 4.2).

The lymph cistern plays a vital role in lymphatic drainage for the lower part of the body, in particular the abdomen and legs, where gravity can hinder lymph circulation. The case studies that follow in the second section of this book will show its significance in conditions as sciatica, low back pain and irritable bowel syndrome. As the lymph enters the subclavian veins and joins with blood, it must go directly to the right side of the heart, then through the capillary beds of the lungs, back to the left side of the heart and then into general circulation. About 20% of the blood goes up into the head, the remainder into the body. Eventually, the filters, i.e. the liver, kidneys, spleen and lungs, must sieve from the blood any toxic matter that remains. If the lymph has not been propelled through lymph nodes to be neutralized, this toxic matter can be significant.

Kidneys

The kidneys filter out toxic amounts of inorganic salts such as sodium chloride, waste products such as uric acid, other metabolic products and the remains of vitamins, hormones, drugs and various chemicals from foods.

The liver

The liver has many lymph vessels and ducts to convey the lymph stream but nevertheless is quickly congested. The many functions of the liver and the receiving of the portal vein with its vast distribution and the hepatic veins collecting and emptying into the vena cava, along the biliary ducts carrying bile into the duodenum, gives an insight into the lymph vessel blockage that can occur if this organ becomes diseased. The hepatic artery supplying the liver has vasomotor regulation and, indirectly, the lymph stream is increased by the normal tone of the artery: The better the blood circulation, the better the lymph

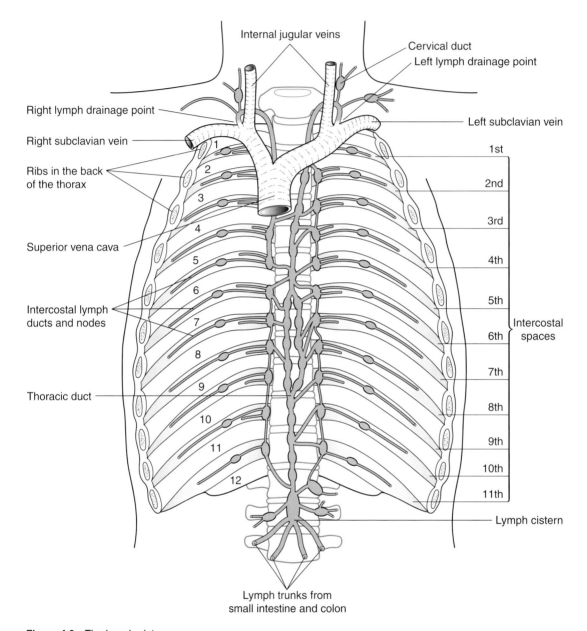

Figure 4.2 The lymph cistern.

flow. Thoracic interference can alter the blood flow to the liver and will cause a slowing down of the lymph through the organ. The left subclavian collects the major part of the liver's lymph; the right lymphatic trunk only part from its convex and posterior surface. It is most important that the left post-clavicular area for thoracic duct drainage is massaged to ensure a healthy liver (Millard 1922).

The spleen and liver

The spleen and liver must filter out excessive fats and proteins as well as metals and minerals.

As the only blood outlet from the spleen is to the liver via the portal vein, all these wastes must eventually be processed and eliminated by the liver. Water-soluble products from the liver return to the bloodstream for elimination by the kidneys; fat solubles enter the bile ductules with bile itself and then pass out of the body via the intestines.

In theory, the lymph should pass through these filters effortlessly. In practice, this is not the case. This is due to three constituents – fibrinogen, white blood cells and chyle – combining together in the lymph to create a glutinous mass.

The constituent of lymph contained in the vessels is dependent on their location (Pickering Pick & Howden 1988). For example, the vessels draining the limbs contain fluid surplus to body needs, which is leaked from cells or blood vessels. This lymph is therefore rich in protein. However, the lymph that is absorbed by the villi of the small intestines is called chyle. Although it resembles lymph in its physical and chemical properties, it has, in addition, a quantity of finely divided fatty particles, which only appear during digestion. Chyle is absorbed by the villi of the small intestine from food and carried by a set of vessels similar to the lymphatics named lacteals, to the left thoracic duct, where it joins the lymph from the lymph cistern and is poured into the circulation (see Fig. 4.1).

Lymph also contains fibrinogen and leukocytes, which clot on removal from the body (Pickering Pick & Howden 1988). It would appear that it is also capable of clotting while still in the body and can adhere to the walls of the lymphatic vessels, causing pockets of congestion. It is this stasis, which does not get filtered by the body, that causes sagging viscera. This restricts nerve impulses controlling not only the circulation but nerve tone, which can be responsible for causing a malfunction in the nervous system.

As was discussed in Chapter 1, every substance produces its own magnetic field – especially this glutinous toxic mass. If this congestion, with its own magnetic field, is in close proximity to a nerve plexus or ganglion, then it is possible that the impulses sent by these junction boxes to the various parts of the body will be distorted.

As the lymph circulates, therefore, it is possible that not all of it will arrive at its destination cleansed of toxic matter. Instead, it can leave toxic residues within the body, in particular the capillaries of the kidneys, spleen and liver, which attract more toxins due to the magnetic field that it creates. To summarize:

1. If the lymph is not flowing freely and is therefore unable to pass through lymph nodes, its toxins will not be neutralized, and the lymphocytes will not increase in number. This vital link essential to our immunity will be impeded (see Chapter 5).
2. If the lymph hasn't been neutralized, as it moves on its journey passing between the lymph and blood capillaries with this glutinous mass, it can adhere in the capillaries, or the lymphatics to vital organs, or the organs themselves, causing problems.
3. Furthermore, if this congestion is sitting close to a nerve plexus, it is possible that the nerve impulses that are directed towards a particular organ are distorted away from their intended destination by the magnetic field of the toxic mass. Therefore those organs will not receive the correct stimulus to function normally.

An understanding of the nervous system is necessary to explain this theory further.

The nervous system

The central nervous system (CNS) consists of billions of interconnecting nerve cells, called neurons, transmitting signals from one part of the nervous system to another.

The sympathetic nervous system controls involuntary activities of the glands, organs, and other parts of the body. This system consists of a series of ganglia (a collection of nerve cells forming a nerve center), connected together by intervening cords. The communications that take place between two or more nerves form what is called a plexus. The abdominal area has many nerve plexuses sending impulses all over the body.

The magnetic field of toxic substances contained within the lymphatics distorts nerve energy and prevents nerve signals from getting to their intended destination. Careful palpation in accessible regions such as the abdomen will reveal this congestion, which if allowed to continue will cause interconnecting energy fields of the body to lose their power resulting in breakdown of communication. An example of this is a stiff neck whose cause often originates in the small intestine (see Chapter 9). (For acupuncture points of the nervous system meridians, see Plan 4B.)

EXERCISE

Any form of activity that can stimulate the lymphatic system is capable of overloading the filters of the body. This applies to all exercise, as the activity of the muscles increases lymphatic flow. It is vital, therefore, that the filters are encouraged to adequately process toxic waste poured into the bloodstream from the lymphatics. Toxins waiting to be disposed of, build up in the bloodstream if the filters are sluggish and the likelihood of toxic matter adhering to tissues and organs after exercise is significant.

The lymphatic system is seldom clear in the normal person. Ever-increasing levels of toxic substances from the environment tax the nodes and vessels at all times. With this in mind, when the lymph passes into the subclavian veins to join with the circulation of blood it goes directly to the right side of the heart, through the capillary beds of the lungs, returning to the left side of the heart before passing into the general circulation. If the lymph has not been detoxified before it is propelled forwards, either during lymphatic drainage or strenuous exercise, it is possible that toxins poured into the blood will stick in the lymphatics of the heart or the heart itself, causing a malfunction.

The sudden death from a heart attack of young, fit healthy individuals following strenuous exercise might actually originate from a congested lymphatic system and inadequate filtering of the liver, kidneys, spleen or lungs. The possibility of lymphatic congestion and even blockage should be investigated in the presence of chest pain. The flow of lymph is as essential as blood and severe congestion is a serious proposition particularly in respect of the heart.

On its website (www.eavnet.com), the International Medical Association for EAV states:

A growing number of patients suffer from chronic illnesses evoked by several different causes as for example: micro-intoxication with pesticides (from food) in addition to a stress imposed to a patient by some varnish in the furniture plus a virus infection that has not been overcome totally. In most of those cases nothing pathological can be found – neither among the laboratory reports nor among other states, ECG and EEG included. Many of those patients, who often have been under examination by quite a number of doctors, are thought to be neurotic or even psychotic. By the measurement with EAV the doctor is able to detect pathologic developments in the organism at an early level, before defects in the structure will result. Several authors hold the opinion that it is possible to make a prevention of degenerative diseases 1 to 2 years before they become visible with usual techniques (ultrasound, X-ray).

FILTER-CLEARING PROCEDURE

It is without question essential to a healthy existence that the filters of the body function to their optimal capacity and that the lymphatic system flows as freely as is possible. Massage to the reflex zones for the liver, kidneys spleen and lungs, and massage into the lymph drainage points above and below the clavicles, is most beneficial before any activity but is vital before receiving *any* therapy including massage or reflexology that promotes the movement of lymphatic fluid

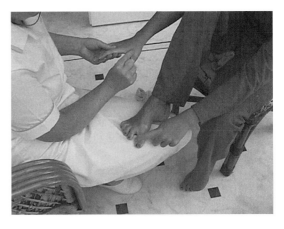

Figure 4.3 ISR liver test.

(see Figs 6.3, p 43 and A2.11a in Appendix 2, p 183). To check that the filters are functioning to their optimum efficiency, acupuncture points related to the filters of the liver, kidneys, spleen and lungs are included in the Plan section. Figure 4.3 shows the ISR test for the liver as an example.

REFERENCES

Millard F P 1922 Applied anatomy of the lymphatics. Australia: International Lymphatic Research Society. (Available from: Health Research, PO Box 850, Pomeroy, Western Australia 99347)
Pickering Pick T, Howden R 1988 Gray's Anatomy (Classic Collector's edition). Crown Publishers, UK, p 1082

5

Why massage is beneficial to lymphatic drainage

Massage, used to encourage lymphatic drainage, is both healing and soothing and an excellent therapy in helping to sustain a healthy body and immune system. Used in conjunction with reflexology and ISR, it is extremely effective.

The skin is the largest organ of the body and contains a good supply of blood, which is brought to the surface by tiny capillaries. Encouraging blood to the surface during massage enables it to pick up waste and toxic substances, depositing them into the lymphatic system for disbursement and allowing fresh lymph to circulate to nourish the tissues.

Lymph contains fibrinogen and leukocytes, which clot on removal from the body. Chyle from the small intestine also contains fibrinogen and the fatty particles from food. These constituents, when contained within the lymphatic fluid, are inclined to congeal but respond very well to massage.

The heat generated when an area of the body is massaged is visible not only by the color of the skin but also by its temperature. This heat helps to dissolve congealed toxins trapped within the lymphatics, thereby allowing ease of flow and thus giving the contents the opportunity to move forward into the lymph nodes, where they can be processed.

The toxic waste discharged into the system for processing after any form of lymphatic drainage is governed by the severity of the congestion and is thereafter dependent upon the efficiency of the lymphatic system for elimination. Few people are in such good health that they have normal lymphatic channels and lymphatic fluid. It is well to remember that any abrasion of the skin (a scratch from a rose thorn, a grazed knee); an abscessed tooth; a diseased tonsil; a sluggish organ, in particular the liver (pain over the right eye); congested areas and glands (for example, cervical or axillary nodes or evidence of edema) are all signs of an irritated and overburdened lymphatic system.

How the lymphatic system works is still not fully understood. Homeopaths provide remedies to assist with lymph drainage; acupuncturists stimulate lymph drainage with needles, moxibustion, electrical impulses and laser; and massage therapists promote lymph clearance from muscle and other tissues, but there is still much to be learned about how the lymphatic system works.

Where treatment of the lymphatic system is given, the treatment might be too superficial, neglecting the deep lymphatics in the abdomen, the neck, under the arms, the intercostal spaces both to the front and at the back of the rib cage, the inguinal nodes, the back of the knees and into the elbows.

Difficulties in assessing problems in the lymphatic system have been the lack of tools for measuring its efficiency, recognition of congestion and the identification of the blocking agents. Observation and palpation are, of course, both necessary and helpful; but inadequate.

The key to objective analysis of the lymphatic system is by way of Voll's acupuncture points directly related to the lymphatic system. Two of the most important points, both on the circulation meridian of the left hand (Ci 8a and Ci 8b) are energetically related to the lymph cistern and thoracic duct, respectively. If a problem is identified on the lymph cistern, then the peritoneum points for the small and large intestines should also be measured to see whether the congestion or overloading extends that far. One of the most frequent causes of complete congestion are transfats from hydrogenated foods, such as some margarines. The higher the proportion of

unsaturated fats in a margarine, the more likely it is that the consumption of that margarine is the cause of the congestion.

Abdominal massage followed by a breathing technique usually clears congestion of the lymph cistern.

EXTRA MERIDIANS

One of the amazing discoveries made by Voll was of eight extra, superficial, non-classical meridians or vessels. These beautifully complement the twelve pairs discovered by the Chinese (Kenyon 1986, p 59). One of the extra pairs is the two lymph vessels that extend from the medial edges of the thumbs up the radial edges of the arms, up over the tops of the shoulders and around the backs of the shoulders to the bladder meridians, connecting with B1 36 (Th 1–2 level). The acupuncture points on the thumb, hand and wrist (Fig. 5.1) are most useful as they can be used to check for lymph drainage problems related to the tonsils, the ears, tubal tonsils, jaw, eyes, sinuses, pharynx, larynx, lungs and heart. Again, massage is one of the best ways of clearing these lymphatics.

The two lymph vessel points Ly 12 and Ly 13 on the front and back edges of the trapezius muscles near the base of the neck are related to problems in the abdominal area and become very tense when there is a stasis in the small intestine. This tension can greatly hinder the flow of lymph from the thoracic duct, which drains into the subclavian vein on the left side, and the flow of lymph from the shorter lymph ducts into the subclavian vein on the right. When there is excessive tension at the nape of the neck it causes excessive tension in the reflex zones in the hands and in the webbing between the thumbs and forefingers, which can easily be tested manually. Numerous substances can cause stasis in the small intestine, including metals that have been excreted from the liver via the bile system and which adhere to the wall of the duodenum at the site of entry from the common bile duct, and which also get trapped in the jejunum. Provided there is some liquid in the duodenum

Figure 5.1 Acupuncture points according to Voll on the palm on the hand. SMP, summation measurement point. The points illustrated are for fingertip testing, assessment, and acupressure only. © F. Fox, used with permission.

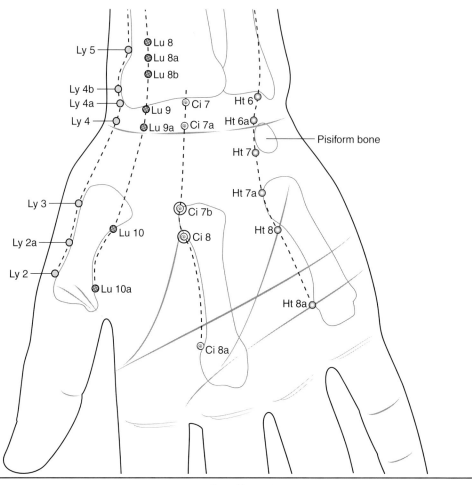

Ly = Lymphatics

Ly 5   –   SMP lymph drainage of heart
Ly 4b –   Larynx and hypopharynx
Ly 4a –   Esophageal drainage
Ly 4   –   Lung drainage
Ly 3   –   Nose and sinuses drainage
Ly 2a –   Eye drainage
Ly 2   –   Teeth; upper and lower jaws drainage

Lu = Lung

Lu 8   –   Veins of the upper extremity
Lu 8a –   Hypopharynx
Lu 8b –   Larynx
Lu 9   –   Trachea
Lu 9a –   Bronchial plexus
Lu 10 –   Bronchi
Lu 10a –   Pleura

Ci = Circulation

Ci 7   –   Coronary artery
Ci 7a –   Coronary plexus
Ci 7b –   SMP lymph systems
Ci 8   –   SMP veins
Ci 8a –   Thoracic duct (accessory or trunk)

Ht = Heart

Ht 6   –   Myocardium
Ht 6a –   Sinus of pericardium
Ht 7   –   Innervation
Ht 7a –   Atrioventricular node
Ht 8   –   Tricuspid valve
Ht 8a –   Pericardium

(ask the patient to drink a glass of water), the congestion can usually be massaged out very quickly (see also Chapter 10). Likewise a congestion in the jejunum. As soon as the congestion is cleared, the muscles in the nape of the neck and the tissues in the webbing of the hands relax (ISR).

Lymphatic drainage in the pelvic area can be tested via the points for the lower hypogastric plexus (B 163) (see Chapter 6 and Plans 2 and 3), as toxic matter trapped in deep lymph nodes usually affects autonomic plexuses and ganglia nearby. Not infrequently, the congestion is a substance trapped in the entrance to the appendix, causing a bad focus. This is a common cause of sciatica and other lower back problems. A disturbance in the inguinal nodes of the right groin could suggest appendix malfunction or disturbance.

the successful removal of metals from the affected area.

The same is true of the parathyroid glands. As these are innervated from the lower cervical ganglia, it is necessary to clear the lymphatics further back at the base of the neck, along the edge of the trapezius muscle each side of the neck, again by using massage. This will help to correct the production of parathormone, which raises the level of calcium in the blood. It can prove to be a great help in solving problems with muscle cramps.

Lymph drainage of the lungs is, of course, of great importance. Overloading of the lung lymphatics usually also blocks the deep acupuncture meridians of the colon, which link the superficial meridians in the front of the shoulders to the transverse colon, right and left. The lung lymphatics can be cleared very easily by tapping the lymph nodes under the intercostal spaces

THE ACUPUNCTURE CONNECTION NEEDS MORE RESEARCH

As toxins in tissue fluid and lymphatic vessels easily block acupuncture meridians, superficial and deep, it is evident that clearance of the lymphatics is of paramount importance to successful acupuncture. It is probable that, once the lymphatics have been cleared, the organs can be tuned via the most basic acupuncture points.

The most obvious example is lymph drainage of the neck along the sternomastoid muscles to clear the nerve supply from the upper and middle cervical ganglia to the thyroid gland (Fig. 5.2). If the lymph nodes in these areas are overloaded with toxic amounts of silver, mercury or cobalt from metals in the mouth, they could either sedate or stimulate the nerve signals to the gland. The production of thyroxin and calcitonin will be affected and no amount of acupuncture will succeed in correcting a problem with basic metabolism or of calcium metabolism. The metals must first be cleared out with massage, and then acupuncture is far more likely to be successful. This can be checked on the endocrine Tw points for the cervical ganglia, End 1a (Fox 1987). After massage, these acupuncture points will confirm

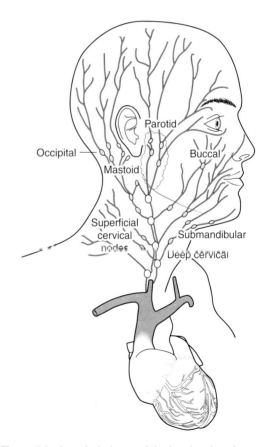

Figure 5.2 Lymph drainage of the head and neck.

both in the front and back of the rib cage. As soon as the congestion is cleared a distinct growl is heard in the abdomen, as the colon reacts to the sudden influx of extra energy via the deep meridian. This is an important exercise for the colon as well as for the lung.

This tapping exercise can also have an effect on the lymph drainage of the heart. In this case it is the small intestine that reacts, and the sound is higher pitched, more like a momentary groan than a growl. These two examples demonstrate the close relationship between the lung and colon, as well as between the heart and the small intestine, well recognized by acupuncture practitioners.

All lymph flows into the bloodstream through two ducts leading into the subclavian veins just before the blood flows into the right auricle of the heart. Elements or chemicals that overload the lymphatics can also become stuck in the endocardium of the heart, both right and left.

This can be checked on acupuncture points (Ht 8b) on the base of the little finger (Fig. 5.3). To clear the endocardium, sharp tapping as in 'do-in' (see pp 33, 179) on the bottom of the sternum is recommended.

The relevance of clearing the lymph drainage of the heart when dealing with edema in the pericardium is evident. However, when dealing with angina and other heart problems its importance is no less. Voll (Voll, personal communication, 1986) stated that lymphatic stasis in the heart is a substantial prerequisite for heart failure in general and for coronary infarct in particular, stases back up into the heart itself, into the myocardium, and around the coronary arteries. Lymphatic pressure against the coronary artery is a frequent cause of angina.

CONTRAINDICATIONS FOR DEEP LYMPH DRAINAGE EXERCISES

1. Overloading of the liver, kidneys, spleen and lungs with toxins or toxic amounts of any substance. However, if such overloading is due to toxins already in lymph nodes near the autonomic ganglia and plexuses that control these organs, those substances must be moved prior to any further drainage. The filters should then be allowed to deal with these substances before more material is transported to them for filtration. In addition, a blockage of the lymph stream

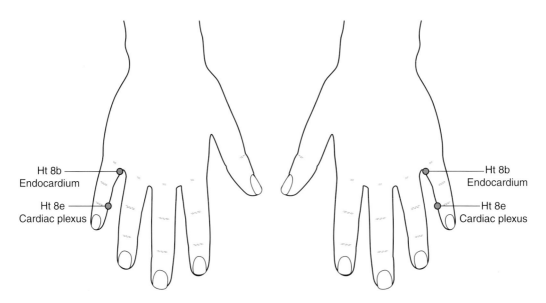

Ht 8b
Endocardium

Ht 8e
Cardiac plexus

Ht 8b
Endocardium

Ht 8e
Cardiac plexus

Figure 5.3 The endocardium and cardiac plexus points (EAV).

at the emptying point of the thoracic duct and right lymphatic duct from possible tension in the muscles of the area will need to be addressed before any lymphatic drainage can begin. For this reason, massage to the area above and below the clavicles followed by reflexology to stimulate the filters is included in all of the case studies. See Fig. A2.11a, p 183.

2. Infectious diseases with raised temperature. The lymphatics should be given time to bring such infections under control and break down the affected matter. Infected matter should never be forced into the bloodstream prematurely because of the risk of blood poisoning.

3. Acute inflammation or fever caused by poisons, bacteria or viruses. Again, because of the danger of blood poisoning, phagocytosis and chelation (binding with protein, especially albumin) should be allowed to take place first.

4. Varicose veins. Massage of the legs is contraindicated, however, the lymphatics should be cleared, as congestion could be restricting venous flow, for example the superficial and deep inguinal nodes. It is wiser to work on the efferents to assist lymph drainage rather than over the actual nodes and abdominal massage could certainly be beneficial. Massage to the reflex zones of the legs should be undertaken.

5. Cancer. Opinion is divided as to the benefits of lymphatic drainage in cancer. Much medical opinion appears to favor the view that cancer is spread via the lymphatic system and infected nodes are duly removed or treated with chemotherapy. However unsure Millard was in 1922, he did state that the liver was the chief organ in systemic pollution and is the primary organ involved, with other organs secondary. If lymphatic drainage is uninhibited there is less chance of malignancy. He believed that the physiological chemistry of the body is dependent upon free-flowing lymph (Millard 1922). The International Medical Association for EAV holds the view that, in the field of prevention by re-establishing the physiological control circuits, cancer could be prevented in 90% of cases, this is according to

scientific indications. This could be achieved by avoiding carcinogenic substances, which are unfortunately on the increase. Laboratory research does not have the means to detect most toxins and therefore EAV will become of interest for those doctors and patients who seek help (www.eavnet.com). Until further research can qualify the benefit of lymphatic drainage in cases of cancer, the condition must be included in the list of contraindications.

SUMMARY

The benefit of a freely flowing lymphatic system and its relationship to the tissues and organs of the body for nourishment and health is very important. Any blockage or congestion in this system must be identified and removed to allow for complete drainage. The webbing of the hand (ATP muscle) acts as an alarm bell in this highly technical early warning system. Its relationship to the immune system (ISR) and its diagnostic value must be taken advantage of if there is to be any progress in the fight against degenerative disease.

This process of lymphatic hygiene forms the basis of therapy.

1. Find the congested areas of the body through fingertip testing and ISR.
2. Identify the cause (possibly a food, food additive or chemical) and exclude it to prevent further blockage.
3. Help the body to eliminate the backlog of toxic fluid through lymphatic drainage, which will enable the body to help itself to recover.
4. Maintain lymphatic hygiene through reflexology, massage and the regular screening of possible allergens through ISR.

A system that has been filtered regularly will not produce much waste, neither will a system that uses the correct food for fuel and avoids using any substances that the body is not able to process.

The filters can be cleared by following the procedures outlined in Chapter 4.

REFERENCES

Fox F 1987 Lymph drainage: an important aid to
acupuncture. Paper presented to the 26th Congress of the
British Acupuncture Association, London; October 16–18
Kenyon J 1986 21st century medicine. Thorsons,
Northampton
Millard F P 1922 Applied anatomy of the lymphatics.
Australia: International Lymphatic Research Society.
(Available from: Health Research, PO Box 850, Pomeroy,
Western Australia 99347)

FURTHER READING

Serizawa K 1976 TSUBO vital points for oriental therapy.
Japan Publications Inc, Tokyo, Japan
Voll R 1982 Measurement points of the electro-
acupuncture according to Voll on the hands and feet
[transl. H Sarkisyanz]. Medizinisch Literarische
Verlagsgesellschaft mbH, Uelzen

The practice of lymphatic drainage

The second section of this book is devoted to actual case studies. It covers massage and the exercises and breathing techniques that encourage lymphatic drainage and alleviate the symptoms presented in each case study. This section explains why it is necessary to practise lymphatic hygiene and describes how this can be achieved. A full explanation of the substances contributing to the symptoms suffered is provided, while at the same time drawing attention to their possible sources. Electro-acupuncture according to Voll (EAV) was used initially to track the route taken in the body by many of these substances and to prove the accuracy of the immune system response (ISR). The relevant reflexology and acupuncture points (for fingertip testing and assessment; not treatment) that are to be used in conjunction with ISR are illustrated at the end of each case study.

Very few patients are in such good health that they have normal, healthy, free-flowing lymphatic fluid, so most are in need of some lymphatic drainage. However, this should be kept simple. Patients should always return home with the ability to clear the filters through reflexology, and a chart emphasizing those areas should be provided together with instructions in performing the relevant exercises (see Plans 1–3). Self-help plays a vital part in lymphatic hygiene. Patients and therapists who would like to use additional reflex zones on the feet relating to specific conditions can do so after following the relevant program.

It is not advisable to use all of the techniques in the book in one session. To achieve maximum benefit from the exercises it is more beneficial to follow them as they are presented for each case study. This will allow the lymph to drain more efficiently and safely. Any drainage exercises should be preceded and finished with massage to the reflex zones on the feet for the liver, kidneys, spleen and lungs, followed by massage above and below the clavicles.

REFLEXOLOGY, CLAVICLE MASSAGE, THE LYMPH CISTERN EXERCISE AND ABDOMINAL MASSAGE

In all of the case studies, the three most important aspects of this lymph drainage technique are reflexology, massage above and below the clavicles, the lymph cistern exercise and abdominal massage.

Reflexology

This ancient art of pressure-point massage was known in India and China 5000 years ago. Reflexology is based on the theory that every organ and system of the body has a corresponding reflex point in the hands and feet. Through reflexology the energy state of any part or system of the body can be tested and treated. This is possible because of the harmonious relationship in energy between them and also because these reflexes are five to twenty times more sensitive than the organs themselves. Reflex points can identify a problem in an organ of the body long before physical symptoms appear. If an organ has not functioned correctly for a period of time, deposits of uric acid crystals or calcium usually form in the reflex points. Until they are reabsorbed, they tend to burden the energy system of the organ involved and hinder its return to normal. Breaking them up and dispersing them through massage hastens the self-healing process. The same applies to hard skin that forms on a reflex point. A callous can be a sign that, in addition to a reduction in the blood supply to the area, perhaps due to pressure of the foot against the shoe, there could also be pressure in the corresponding organ. The removal of both the hard dead skin and the deposits of uric acid crystals speed recovery to the corresponding organ (Berkson 1977).

Reflexology points on the feet are very responsive and for this reason these zones are featured in the case studies.

The best position for reflexology is with the patient lying flat with the head supported by a pillow. For treatment at home, a relaxed position for both the recipient and the person who is administering the therapy is important. Lying on the floor, with the leg elevated on the other person's lap, is acceptable. Additive-free cream or almond oil on the pad of the thumb can be used (provided an allergic reaction to nuts is not a problem). Massage should be firm and in a circular motion to the areas that are marked on the patient's chart. If there is not another person to help with the massage then a golf ball, with the foot

(a)

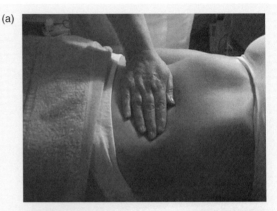

(b)

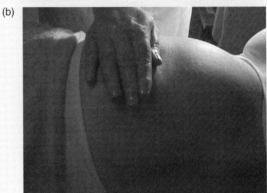

Figure S2.1   Therapist lymph drainage (Exercise 1).

placed on top, can be rolled on the floor allowing the appropriate point to be massaged gently.

Massage above and below the clavicles

Massage into the tissues above and below the clavicles (see Fig. A2.11a in Appendix 2).

Lymph cistern exercise

This exercise should always be performed after reflexology. The lymph cistern is protected by the abdominal aorta but it is the ducts leading to the cistern that are subject to compression and blockage by gastric pressure. The following exercise clears the cistern very well.

Place both hands over the abdomen by the navel and ask the patient to push out the abdomen against your hands without breathing in (Fig. S2.1). Ask the patient to breathe in deeply while maintaining the pressure and even increasing it for a short time before relaxing and exhaling. Repeat three times.

Ensure that pressure exerted is directed to the hands on the navel. The patient must not direct any pressure to the head.

The cistern

The cistern, which is located at the level of the second lumbar vertebra just in front of the aortic artery and vein, has to be clear to allow vitamin D, which is fat soluble, to be absorbed in the chyme from the intestines. An important vitamin, it is required by the body to regulate the balance of calcium and phosphate and to aid the absorption of calcium from the intestine; it is essential for strong bones and teeth. Although too much vitamin D is harmful, can lead to abnormal calcium deposits in the soft tissues and is detrimental for people with arthritis, it is still needed by the body. Diet is by far the best way of receiving vitamin D; oily fish (such as sardines, herring, salmon and tuna), liver and egg yolk all contain this vitamin. In the body, vitamin D is formed by the action of ultraviolet rays in sunlight on a specific chemical in the skin. If sun therefore doesn't cause the patient a problem, it could be beneficial in small doses.

Abdominal massage

In all of the case studies in this section, abdominal massage is given for the following reason: The duodenum is the first part of the small intestine, extending from the lower end of the stomach to the boundary of the jejunum. Ducts from the pancreas, liver and gallbladder feed into the duodenum and a malfunction could quickly develop in these organs if the nerve supply to the duodenum is blocked or interrupted. A spasm in the duodenum disrupts the energy to the abdominal muscles, which in turn causes them to go into spasm. This restricts the nerve supply to and from all the ganglia and plexuses (which are plentiful in the abdominal region) and can cause a knock-on effect to almost every area of the body. Abdominal massage *always* removes the spasm from the duodenum and plays an important role in this lymphatic drainage technique.

Massage technique

The patient's comfort and dignity must always be of prime consideration in abdominal massage. It is vital to help the patient relax during this treatment, therefore only the abdomen should be exposed. It is also important that the lubricant used is acceptable to the patient's immune system. Using ISR can help to assess this.

Begin by gently palpating the abdomen to relax the patient, who might feel discomfort due to congestion. As the muscles relax the therapist can then proceed with massage, being aware at all times of areas of sensitivity.

Massage should proceed with small, gentle, circular movements in the region of the ascending colon in a clockwise direction. Work towards the hepatic flexure, concentrating on this area for several minutes before moving on across the transverse colon into the splenic flexure, focusing here again for several minutes. This process must continue until the tissue feels relaxed.

At this stage, the pressure of massage should deepen, whereupon increased penetration should focus on the appendix/cecum area working into and under the anterior superior iliac spine for some minutes (providing the patient does not feel any discomfort). Continue in this vein while moving up through the colon to the left side and down into the sigmoid colon, where massage should again be sustained for a few minutes. At this stage, move to the small intestine and continue with small circular movements again for a few minutes.

This process must continue for approximately 20 minutes.

Abdominal massage given by a trained therapist is obviously the preferred method, but the simplified version of self-help abdominal massage presented below is quite adequate when done correctly. It is not advisable for an untrained person to attempt a full abdominal massage on an elderly patient because of the location of the aorta in respect of the area being massaged. There must also be an awareness of the possibility of osteoporosis when working around the rib cage.

Self-help abdominal massage

Sitting in a chair with the back supported, the patient should follow the line of the rib cage with the fingers, gently massaging the soft tissue just beneath (Fig. S2.2). Doing this several times, increasing the depth of the massage, will relax any spasm that has formed in the duodenum. Taking the left hand the patient should cross it over the abdomen and push the fingers into the appendix area, holding the right hand over the left to exert a little pressure. Tensing the abdominal muscles, push the abdomen out against the fingers and hold for 5 seconds. This should be repeated on the left side. The patient should then return to the rib cage and massage again with the fingers. This form of abdominal massage will help to stimulate many of the nerves in the abdominal region and the patient will gain enormous benefit by performing this one massage alone.

Do-in

This is a therapy used often by the Chinese as an ancient art of self-massage using gentle poundings and finger pressure to equalize and restore the energy circulating within the body. The advantage of do-in is that it can be performed

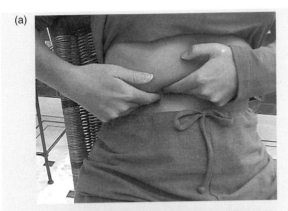

(a)

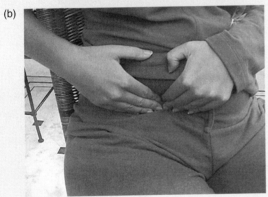

(b)

Figure S2.2 Self-help abdominal massage.

by the patient to assist the lymph to move through the vessels (Fig. A2.3 on p 179).

By flexing the wrist and forming a loose weak fist with the hand enables the pounding of these areas to be performed effortlessly (de Langre 1980).

Caution

People with diabetes who would like to use these lymphatic drainage techniques should monitor their blood sugar levels carefully after the program. The stimulation of nerve plexuses to the pancreas together with the stimulus gained through the reflex points for the liver can improve insulin absorption.

All patients should be prepared for a lowering in body temperature within half an hour of completing the lymphatic drainage exercises for the first time. To help the body to eliminate this extra burden of waste as efficiently as possible, it is advisable to ask the patient to drink at least eight glasses of water a day for 3 days following a treatment session. This will not only assist the liver and kidneys but will limit the effects of the cleansing process. This could include diarrhea, headache or even mouth ulcers for a short time until the benefits of the techniques are experienced.

REFERENCES

Berkson D 1977 The foot book. Harper and Row, New York
de Langre J 1980 The first book of do-in. Happiness Press, California

6

Back pain

FIRST VISIT

When Stephen stepped into the clinic in August 1990 and asked for help it was very obvious that he was in pain. He had suffered from lower back pain for almost 5 years but over the last 18 months the pain had increased in intensity and had spread to his upper spine and right arm. At about the time this latest discomfort started, he suffered an acute attack of heartburn with a burning sensation to his throat and stomach. He said that he felt as though this whole area was on fire.

Stephen saw his doctor with regard to these latest developments, which resulted in intensive hospital tests. The medical investigations revealed inflammation of the stomach and esophagus, and arthritis (in its early stages) of the spine.

Stephen was taking a combination of drugs, which included anti-inflammatories, analgesics and drugs to combat the acid in his stomach.

Stephen was only 41 but his deteriorating health meant that his quality of life was poor. Rather than being eased by the medication, his symptoms appeared to be intensifying, and he was becoming more dependent on painkillers for his back pain, which he felt aggravated his stomach. He was an enthusiastic gardener but he was now unable to cope with many tasks in the garden and felt it was only a matter of time before he would have to employ help or move house. His job entailed a considerable amount of driving around the country but his back condition was limiting the amount of time he could spend at the wheel. He had to make frequent stops to try and relieve the discomfort, especially on long journeys. The situation was becoming intolerable, so his doctor had suggested that further investigations were necessary and had referred him to a consultant.

Spinal X-rays had not revealed any bone abnormality or been otherwise conclusive. Stephen's consultant suggested a course of physiotherapy over a 6-week period. However this had to be abandoned after 3 weeks because of increased pain. Manipulation under anesthetic followed, which also proved fruitless, as did acupuncture, which was so painful that his whole back went into spasm during the first session. His consultant felt that the only alternative was an exploratory operation. Stephen's attitude was that he would rather avoid this drastic probing and he asked for more time to consider the implications attached to such measures.

The causes behind back pain are often not fully understood. Tests, including X-rays are often inconclusive: they cannot prove that back pain is attributed to a serious underlying condition. The back presents more of a problem to doctors than any other area. Disabling low back pain strikes 80% of us during our lifetimes, causes millions of lost work days and is second only to head pain in patients seeking help from their general practitioners. Unfortunately, doctors seem no nearer to understanding back pain than they ever were, despite endless research into its diagnosis, causes and treatment. It would appear that misdiagnosis or unproven and aggressive treatment with drugs and surgery contribute more to the problems of back pain sufferers than they do to the solutions (Thomas 1999).

A leading expert on the subject, Professor Gordon Waddell, has suggested that most surgical procedures prove fruitless and, indeed, as few as 1% of patients who undergo surgery for lumbar disorders enjoy success: in the 99% of patients complaining of simple backache, the problem becomes worse, despite investigations and treatments (Thomas 1999).

There are occasions, of course, when back conditions originate from mechanical disorders such as ruptured or herniated discs or deteriorating vertebrae. However, the vast majority of chronic back pain sufferers do not find the cause of their symptoms and therefore are not able to alleviate them: Traditional methods of diagnosis are evidently ineffective as chronic low back pain continues to be common, expensive and difficult to manage by traditional medical and surgical treatment (Thomas 1999).

In situations where investigative surgery appears to be the only way to form a diagnosis, complementary therapy has very good results. In particular, a therapy that can establish an incomplete or low energy magnetic field within the body, suggesting lymphatic congestion. The negative energetic interactions between congested lymph nodes and nerve plexuses quickly lead to physiological faults that can be difficult to identify by any other means. If permanent damage of the spine is to be avoided, the exact location of the congestion should be identified as quickly as possible. To do so is the first positive step towards the healing process.

Stephen was a conscientious man with three children. He could see a good future for himself in his present company and he very much wished to continue working.

Stephen was taken through a range of movements to assess the flexibility of his spine.

There was an obvious restriction in the lower spine, which had been confirmed by his consultant. Using EAV, Stephen's acupuncture points were tested and in the points that registered a low reading, formaldehyde and substances contained within medication, similar to that which Stephen was taking were identified. These areas of congestion were the upper mesenteric plexus, the upper and lower hypogastric plexus and the celiac plexus. The kidneys, liver, pancreas, stomach and small and large intestines were also reading very low in energy, suggesting congestion of these areas too.

Patient participation is extremely important in this type of therapy because it is necessary to identify the source of the contamination in the hope that it can be eliminated from the patient's environment, which in Stephen's case was formaldehyde and medication. Unfortunately, this is not always an easy task, lymphatic congestion can be the result of years of accumulation; the source then becomes difficult to determine.

According to Collins English Dictionary, formaldehyde has a pungent, characteristic odor. It is found in: traffic fumes, glues and cements, matches, cigarettes, candle wicks, foam rubber, furniture, pillows, mattresses, carpets, fabric softeners, orthopedic casts, surgical instrument cleaning materials, dyes, permanent press treatment, mildew proofing, medium density fiberboard (MDF) (especially when cut), water-repellent treatment, moth proofing, antiperspirants, antiseptics, paper manufacture, newspaper print, copying machines, tanned animal skins, germicidal soaps, detergents, fungicides, insecticides, some shampoos and hair-setting lotion, nail polish, air deodorants, concrete, plaster, wallboard, synthetic resins, wood veneers, wood preservatives and cavity wall insulation. It is also used in the manufacturing process of vitamins A and E and in the manufacture of some antibiotics.

There is evidence that some people can develop a sensitivity to formaldehyde. Even in small amounts, formaldehyde can cause serious health problems and, according to the findings, it takes years to dissipate after being used in manufactured products.[1] In some cases, exposure to formaldehyde can increase a person's sensitivity to other irritants or chemicals that were never a problem in the past, making them allergic to almost anything. It has also been shown to cause cancer in animals and might cause cancer in humans (Environmental Protection Agency).

The antidote to formaldehyde is vinegar. Patients who are having difficulty eliminating formaldehyde from their systems should tape some cotton wool soaked in vinegar to their forearm for 3 days. The magnetic field of the vinegar will cancel the antagonistic magnetic field of formaldehyde. This can be tested using ISR.

A potential cause of cancer (Allergy Newsletter 1997)

[MDF], the material which many give a home to in kitchen units, wardrobes and bookcases, may be a cancer risk, especially in poorly ventilated houses. When it is cut, drilled or sanded, it releases fine dust coated with formaldehyde, a potential cause of lung cancer and nose and throat cancer, according to Dr Andrew Watterson, director of the Centre for Occupational and Environmental Health, Leicester.
(Allergy Newsletter 1997)

Identifying the source of Stephen's congestion with formaldehyde was not easy, with so many sources of contact. The most obvious source of contact was the fabric conditioner used in the washing machine.

Stephen's congestion was not only caused by formaldehyde but also by the cocktail of drugs he was taking. Patients are frequently told that they need to take these drugs to relieve their symptoms. However, the actual cause of the problem can become hidden amidst the ever-increasing congestion of chemicals that are contained within drugs. Very often, simple lymphatic drainage techniques are all that is required to relieve severe pain after the congested areas have been identified. (Care should be taken if patients decide to reduce their

medication and such reduction should be done in consultation with their GP.)

The vast majority of people with lower back problems also suffer from constipation, the most common cause of which is painkillers. Constipation occurs due to congested lymphatics in the region of sympathetic nerve plexuses, especially the lower and upper hypogastric plexuses that energize the intestines and rectum. This was confirmed in Stephen's case on testing the acupuncture points for the plexuses and identification of the medication that Stephen was taking.

When these plexuses register a low energy, the impulses from the nerves to stimulate the bowel to empty are not strong enough to perform this function. Constipation is the result and laxatives are often prescribed. However, laxatives override the struggling nerve supply and directly stimulate the bowel to contract. This is acceptable in the short term, or for emergencies, but if the situation continues for any length of time it will be difficult to restore normal nerve function and stimulus to those muscles that perform the task of defecation naturally. Equally, enlarged and overburdened lymph nodes and vessels in the pelvic cavity will undoubtedly put enormous stress on the transverse colon and can cause it to sag. Once an organ or tissue alters position in the pelvic region, the mesentery misaligns and this leads to negative intercommunications between the nerve plexus and tissues of the entire pelvic cavity. This results in very weak peristalsis and muscle function. Unless the decongestion within the abdominal and pelvic lymphatics and organs has been addressed, the likelihood of any back condition responding to treatment on a permanent basis is slim. The particular lymphatic drainage exercises outlined in the treatment section help to reverse this stasis and the natural function of the bowel, but if constipation lasts for more than a week a doctor should be consulted as a more serious condition might be the cause.

The upper hypogastric plexus
This is the nerve station that supplies the pelvic cavity and many organs within, including the

---

[1] The Environmental Protection Agency (EPA) has developed the Healthy Home Test Kit, which measures concentrations of formaldehyde. This kit is easy to use and comes with complete instructions. See Appendix 3: list of suppliers for details.

appendix, cecum, upper right colon, duodenum and descending colon. It is situated in front of the sacrum, between the iliac arteries.

Whenever the energy to this point is low, the colon is invariably highly congested with toxins and the patient will undoubtedly be suffering from low back pain. A spasm can usually be identified in the region of lumbar 4 and 5. (This will respond to back massage, although this response will remain cosmetic if the nerve supply to the plexus is not corrected first.) The organs in the pelvic cavity are highly vulnerable if congested lymph nodes and vessels are responsible for distorted energy. This vulnerability stems not only from their lack of stimuli but also from the muscles and ligaments attached to the innominate bones as they spasm and misalign, causing an unevenness of the cavity. With little space in the cavity, any small movement is noticed and organs can be squeezed together, which could badly affect their blood supply and further result in lymphatic stasis. Particular victims of this congestion are the sacroiliac ligaments and joints, which weaken and cause sagging of the pelvis. This throws the legs and hips out of line and the strain is often felt in the knees.

The psoas muscles too are usually badly affected and will spasm; this will exacerbate pain by causing a misalignment of the spine as the ilium rotates anterior or posterior. These all-important psoas muscles when in spasm, cannot help but affect the structures and organs in the region.

These are the knock-on effects of congestion of the lymphatics and failing communication system in the abdominal/pelvic region. This vicious circle of events will gather momentum and the joints that are so dependent upon these structures for their support and strength will be unable to endure the strain. The patient's condition will deteriorate further unless organs, muscles and tendons in the abdomen and pelvis retain their tone and respective locality and this cannot be brought about by administering more drugs, and more chemicals, and so producing even more congestion!

Psoas muscles

These muscles are primary hip flexors. They consist of two parts: psoas major and psoas minor, which originate from the lower spine. The lower end of the psoas minor is attached to the pelvis, and the lower end of the psoas major is attached to just below the neck of the femur. The strain on these bones caused by the muscles in spasm will inevitably result in the symptoms displayed by Stephen. Eventually, if these muscles stay in this permanent state, hip problems will develop and will become another symptom of incorrect nerve stimuli causing physiological faults (Fig. 6.1).

The sacroiliac joint

This is an articulation between the sacrum and the ilium on each side of the body. The bony surfaces within the joint are lined with cartilage and have a small amount of synovial fluid between them. Strong ligaments between the sacrum and ilium permit only minimal movement at the joint. The sacroiliac joint can be strained, usually as a result of childbirth or repetitive stress involved in sports such as athletics due to overstriding. Discomfort is felt over the sacroiliac

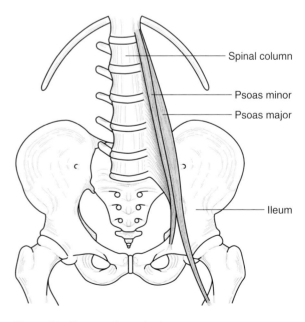

Figure 6.1   Psoas major and minor.

joint, the buttock to the thigh and leg, and very often the groin. Indeed, this joint can be the cause of many back problems, yet, unfortunately, it is not identified by X-ray (British Medical Association 1990, see also Hutson 1990).

As shown in Fig. 6.2, the sacroiliac joint is not in a prominent position and its stability is often misunderstood. It is commonly thought that this joint is affected only by bone, muscle and ligament structures, whereas it is also affected by the lymphatic connection and abdominal congestion, and these should be considered when treating lower back pain or associated sacroiliac joint problems.

The severe pain that sears down the leg from the lower spine – often called sciatica – also originates in the abdomen. The sciatic nerve passes below the sacroiliac joint and backwards to the buttock, from where it passes behind the hip joint and runs down the back of the thigh. A misaligned sacroiliac joint and rigid muscles are responsible for trapping the nerve and causing the searing pain. The weakened pelvic muscles and ligaments (in particular the broad ligaments, which support the pelvic organs) can also be a major factor in gynecological and bladder problems.

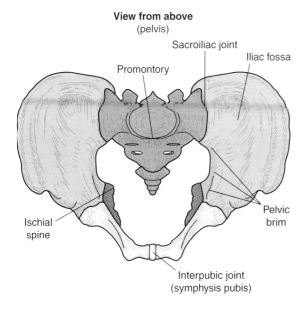

View from above
(pelvis)

Sacroiliac joint

Iliac fossa

Promontory

Pelvic brim

Ischial spine

Interpubic joint
(symphysis pubis)

Figure 6.2   The sacroiliac joint.

The exercises in the treatment section will help to clear the lower lymphatics, and encourage the oscillations needed for precise electrical activity between nerve plexuses and tissues. The resulting muscle and ligament stimulation of the pelvic area will be beneficial for the majority of back conditions. In addition, women of all ages who wish to retain pelvic muscle control would be well advised to follow these exercises to limit the incidence of incontinence during the menopause and in later life.

The mesenteric plexus
This is located just behind the base of the pancreas and stimulates the small intestine, colon and rectum. The nerves intertwine just below the transverse colon. Abdominal massage is involved in the decongesting of the lymphatics relating to both the mesenteric and celiac plexuses.

The celiac plexus
This is located close to the diaphragm and is the nerve supply to the pancreas that controls the production of enzymes. If faulty, it can result in food sensitivities because the enzymes that are needed to digest food will not be produced. It subdivides into the gastric, hepatic and splenic plexuses. The gastric plexus is the main nerve supply to the stomach. Congestion of the lymphatics in this area can not only result in food sensitivities but also in stomach problems. The lymph drainage exercises and massage in the treatment section are designed to drain the vessels and nodes to the areas surrounding the above plexuses.

Treatment

Therapists and patients alike will have no difficulty working from the photographs in Appendices 1 and 2. The treatment procedure will be exactly the same in either case. However, should any pain or difficulty be experienced in executing any of the breathing techniques or exercises then these should not be continued, rather move on to the next exercise. Return to the exercises which have caused difficulty when a few days have elapsed, providing that any procedure is concluded with the reflexology zones for the liver, kidneys, spleen and lungs.

Full details of how to perform the exercises in the following list can be found in Appendix 1.

1. Reflexology. It is very important that the filtering system of the body is functioning to its optimal efficiency prior to any lymph drainage exercises. Equally important are the two lymph drainage points in the supraclavicular regions. If congestion is evident here (identifiable by puffiness or tenderness) then correct lymphatic drainage of other areas will not be successful. For this reason the following two exercises are crucial to the success of the therapy program:

(i) reflexology to the liver, kidneys, spleen, lungs and subclavian lymph drainage points of both feet (see Fig. 6.3, pp 43–44)

(ii) massage above and below the clavicles.

2. Exercise 1, Lymph cistern.

3. Abdominal massage. The benefit of this massage cannot be exaggerated. The draining of the lymphatics of the abdomen is invaluable to the many nerve plexuses and ganglia in the abdominal region, and never more so than for back pain. On the first treatment, Stephen's abdomen was very tender. This is due not only to the lack of muscle tone but also to the lack of complete lymphatic drainage in the abdominal region. This discomfort is noticeable upon palpation of the abdomen for the first time. However, it should ease once the nerve supplies have been stimulated and the drainage becomes more effective. This massage is certainly beneficial where constipation is a problem.

4. Foot rotation. This exercise activates the nerves that supply energy to the muscles and ligaments of the pelvis. This helps to release any constraint to the sciatic nerve and, combined with Exercise 3 (inguinal drain), is very successful for pelvic and lower back conditions.

Foot rotation and Exercise 3 (inguinal drain) combined with reflexology, lymph drainage point massage, Exercise 1 (lymph cistern) and do-in, would be beneficial prior to any long-haul flight.

Foot rotation can then continue during the flight at half-hour intervals.

5. Exercise 3, inguinal drain. This exercise clears the lymphatics of the small intestine and colon as well as the areas around the rectum.

6. Repeat Exercise 1, lymph cistern.

7. Do-in. This is a therapy used by the Chinese. An explanation is given on p 33. Many of the case histories will require the patient to perform this simple but effective technique to particular areas of the body at a precise point in the therapy program. (This must not be performed if there is a problem with brittle bones.) For this treatment program tap gently either side of the sternum.

8. Reflexology. To the liver, kidney, spleen lungs, pancreas, sacroiliac joint, psoas muscle, lymph cistern and subclavian lymph drainage points. This will conclude the exercise program (see Fig. 6.3, pp 43–44).

It would be advisable for the patient to repeat the program once a day for 2 weeks followed by alternate days until symptoms subside.[2] Thereafter, repeat once or twice a week as a lymphatic maintenance regime. As an extra helping hand to assist the body in its removal of the toxins, it is recommended that the patient drink eight glasses of water a day for 3 days.

After the above exercises, Stephen's acupuncture points relating to the nerve plexuses mentioned above were not 100% but they had all improved. He returned home with a chart for reflexology, notes on the exercises and instructions to drink eight glasses of water a day for the next 3 days.

SECOND VISIT

Three weeks later, Stephen returned with the information on the source of his formaldahyde. It was highly probable that a well-known antibacterial cleanser he used to clean his greenhouse each year and the wood preservative that he used to protect the garden fence were the

---

[2] Appendix 2 contains instructions to the patient on how to perform the exercises in Appendix 1.

source of contact. He did not wear protective gloves while carrying out either of these jobs and also possessed a liking for their smell, which he inhaled freely. Cleaning the greenhouse was usually performed when it was a sunny, but cold day; therefore the greenhouse door was invariably closed.

Identifying this source of contact was most significant and answered my many questions as to the reason why Stephen's body appeared to be so congested with this chemical. The rate at which formaldehyde is released from products is accelerated by heat and can also depend on the humidity level. Formaldehyde tends to double its level of outgassing for every 10°F increase in temperature, which is pertinent when working in a greenhouse.

Adequate protection must be given to the body when performing jobs of this nature, to prevent any penetration of potentially harmful chemicals. Gloves are a must, and also a mask to cover the nose and mouth and prevent the fumes from entering the nasal cavity and the lungs. The use of dehumidifiers and air conditioning to control humidity and maintain a moderate temperature is recommended to help reduce emissions from any product containing formaldehyde.

This second visit Stephen said his back condition was different. The whole of his back felt badly bruised and was uncomfortable, especially in bed. Movement, was easier and so he felt confident that the treatment was doing something. He had reduced his painkillers and felt clear-headed. I suspected a frozen shoulder was the reason for pain and limited movement to the right arm. This would be considered at a later date. The second treatment continued in much the same vein as the first but with the inclusion of Exercise 4 (the four-step exercise).

Treatment

Follow the treatment procedure:

1. **Reflexology and massage to drainage points.**
2. **Exercise 1, lymph cistern.**
3. **Abdominal massage.**
4. **Foot rotation.**
5. **Exercise 3, inguinal drain.**
6. **Exercise 4, the four-step exercise.** This exercise helps to stimulate the nerve supplies of the celiac plexus (abdominal aortic plexus, solar plexus, duodenum and jejunum) and decongests the superior mesenteric lymph nodes in the epigastrium. It is best performed by the patient under the guidance of the therapist and can be repeated at home.
7. **Do-in.** Tap gently either side of the sternum.
8. **Reflexology.** To the liver, kidney, spleen, lungs, pancreas, sacroiliac joint, psoas muscles, lymph cistern and drainage points. This will conclude the exercise program (see Fig. 6.3, pp 43–44).

THIRD VISIT

After 3 weeks a more hopeful man walked into the clinic. Stephen's lower back had improved dramatically, but he was very wary of triggering the whole process off again and was afraid of overdoing anything. The reading for the vast majority of acupuncture points had returned to normal. Stephen was reassured that gentle exercise was necessary to improve the tone of the muscles, in particular the lower spine, now that the energy to and from the nerve plexuses had been restored. Any exercise that requires the patient on all fours such as washing the kitchen floor is of great benefit – the twisting movement from side to side can be very useful in helping to keep the spine spasm free.

Stephen was responding very well to the treatment and continuing the exercises and massaging the reflex zones at home.

His right arm was only marginally better but, when questioned about his stomach, he was surprised at the level of improvement. With the agreement of his doctor his medication had been reduced further, not only for the back problem but also for his stomach, which was not producing anywhere near the original amount of acid prior to the treatments.

Stephen's consultant had been interested to hear of the improvement to his spine when he attended the hospital at his last appointment.

The consultant also confirmed the diagnosis that he was indeed suffering from a frozen shoulder. Cortisone injections were suggested by the consultant for the condition if it didn't improve.

Stephen's back condition continued its pattern of improvement and, within 3 months, he was free from the searing pain that he had previously experienced and he maintained the improvement using the techniques outlined in the case study at home.

Stephen did not need to move house or employ help in the garden and he has been promoted in his job and is very happy with his level of fitness. There are occasions, however, when he is reminded of the pain. This usually occurs after he has lifted something heavy and has forgotten to do his exercises for a few months. He is able to rectify the situation quickly by returning to his exercise regime.

Stephen was tested for food sensitivity, and was found to be intolerant to tea, milk, wheat and coffee. By avoiding these foods his stomach problems and frozen shoulder greatly improved. His case study is continued in Chapter 10.

The reflexology charts and acupuncture points that are relevant for this case study are shown in Figs 6.3 and 6.4 and are to be used in conjunction with ISR and lymphatic drainage techniques. Practising lymphatic hygiene in this way should assist the body in avoiding physiological dysfunction thus attaining structural alignment and the prevention of degenerative disease.

REFERENCES

Allergy Newsletter 1997 Number 61, Winter issue, p 27
British Medical Association 1990 Complete family health encyclopaedia. Dorling Kindersley, London
Collins English Dictionary (3rd edn) 1991 HarperCollins, London
Environmental Protection Agency (EPA). Formaldehyde. Online. Available: http://www.prohousedr.com/epa%20formaldehyde.htm
Thomas P 1999 Back pain: the curve ball symptom. What doctors don't tell you. 1999; 10(5) August

FURTHER READING

Hutson M A 1990 Sports injuries. Oxford University Press, Oxford
McKenzie R 1981 The lumbar spine: mechanical diagnosis and therapy. Spinal Publications, New Zealand
Oliver J 1999 Back in line. Butterworth-Heinemann, London
Reed Gibson P 2000 Multiple chemical sensitivity. New Harbinger Publications Inc, Oakland, California
Waddell G 1998 The back pain revolution. Churchill Livingstone, Edinburgh
Wiesel S W, Weistein J N, Herkowitz H, Bell G (eds) 1990 The lumbar spine. W B Saunders, Philadelphia

Right foot

Left foot

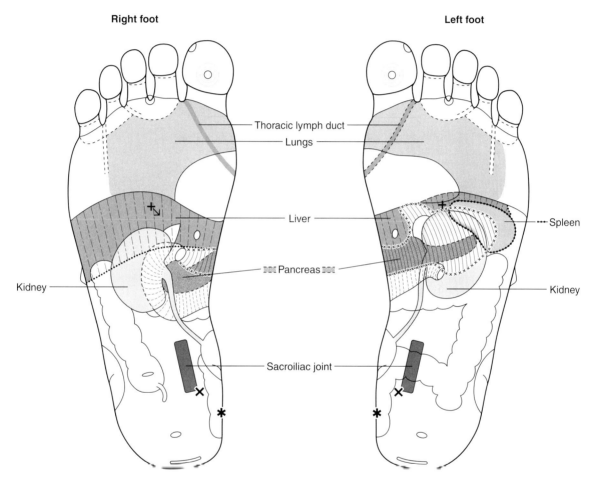

Thoracic lymph duct

Lungs

Liver

Spleen

Pancreas

Kidney

Kidney

Sacroiliac joint

Figure 6.3   Reflexology chart for the liver, kidneys, spleen, lungs, pancreas, sacroiliac joint, psoas muscle, lymph cistern and subclavian lymph drainage points of both feet. © F. Fox, used with permission.

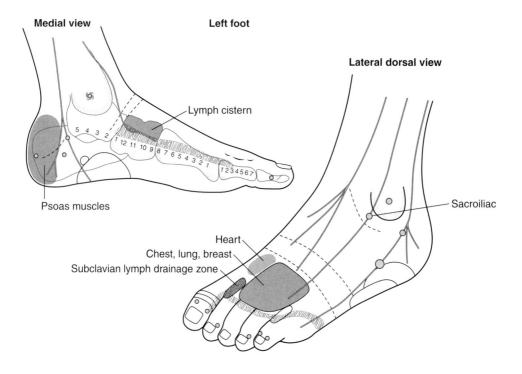

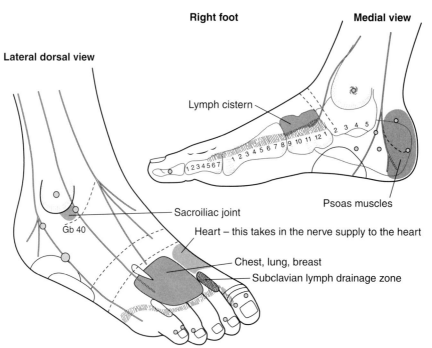

Figure 6.3 *(continued)*.

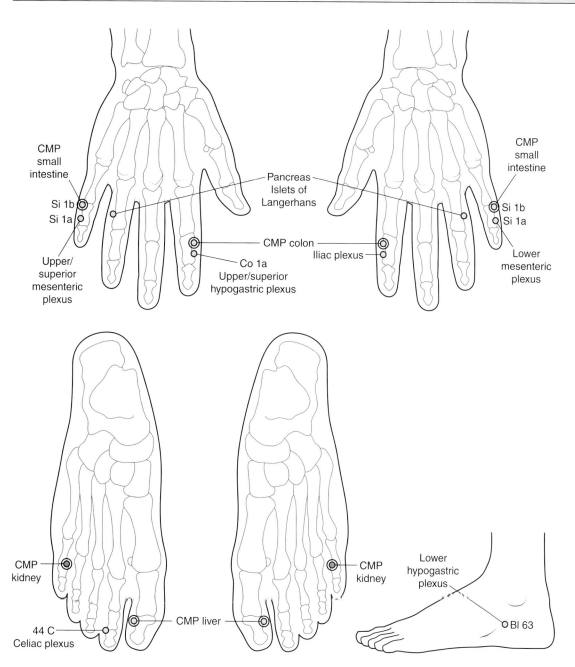

Figure 6.4   Relevant acupuncture points on the hands and feet. The points illustrated are for fingertip testing and assessment, and not for treatment. CMP, control measurement point.

7

Irritable bowel syndrome and an unexpected breast abnormality

FIRST VISIT

Jean, 61, had been diagnosed with irritable bowel syndrome (IBS) many years previously but the condition had become unbearable in the last 3 months. The pain had increased and the bouts of diarrhea meant that she was virtually confined to her home. Alarmed at the sudden change in her symptoms, Jean attended her local hospital where investigations had proved inconclusive.

This condition, which affects a large percentage of the population, is a combination of intermittent abdominal pain and irregular bowel habit (i.e. constipation, diarrhea or bouts of each). Food sensitivities can be the cause behind these debilitating symptoms and often an allergic reaction to gluten is the problem. If this is the case then clearly the offending food substances must be removed from the patient's diet and this can produce remarkable results. Patients who suffer from chronic sinus problems are amazed how suddenly these symptoms disappear too. Sinus problems and the mucus that is produced can quite often be the first sign of food sensitivity and can precede any bowel problems. Mucus-laden diarrhea is fairly common in patients who suffer from food intolerance, particularly if milk is the offending food. When the body receives food that it doesn't particularly like it tries to get rid of it as quickly as possible. This agitation causes increased bowel peristalsis, which irritates the wall of the bowel,

producing mucus in the stool and/or diarrhea. High-fiber breakfast cereals can also have a similar effect, so do bear this in mind. Food sensitivities need to be identified but very often the underlying cause is not established. The situation can become chronic resulting in further food sensitivities, tiredness and much distress.

On testing Jean's acupuncture points, black dye was evident in most of the plexuses associated with the intestines: the mesenteric plexuses, the hypogastric plexus and also the celiac plexus, which energizes the pancreas. The mediastinal plexus, a minute plexus beneath the pleura that stimulates the alveoli, the tiny sacs in the lungs involved with the oxygen/carbon dioxide exchange, had a similarly low reading. Judging by the low output reading for the left kidney, it too was heavily overburdened by the elimination of black dye.

Over the years it has become apparent that when the celiac plexus has a low energy reading, food sensitivities are a major contributing factor in the symptoms presented by the patient. In my experience, any patient who is seriously congested will develop a sensitivity to almost all foods. It is therefore prudent for the majority of patients to wait a while for their system to clear before testing for food sensitivity. There are exceptions, however, and these will be discussed in later chapters. As Jean's acupuncture readings were not too low, she would benefit from avoiding those foods that her body wasn't really happy with.

The substances to which Jean was intolerant included:

- Milk and its by-products (cream, ice cream, yogurt, cheese, etc.) cakes, potato and wheat.
- Black dye: this substance appears regularly in the lymphatics of patients who suffer from bowel disturbances. Carbon from newsprint is another substance and, quite remarkably, the two appear to have very similar magnetic fields, which can often make it difficult to differentiate between them.
- Black leather footwear: always registers high on the list of possible sources of contact when black dye is established in an area of the body. This permeation happens especially if the shoes become wet either through rain, or perspiration. The dye can often be seen on the feet, even though socks or tights have been worn, and it can travel from the feet to the intestines via the lymphatic system, which is exactly what happened to Jean.
- Black leather belts: another source of contact that can affect the intestines, particularly the transverse colon. The dye can be absorbed through the skin of the waist area, where it will distort nerve impulses from the many ganglia in the abdominal and thoracic regions.

Jean apparently always wore black leather shoes and gloves, but rarely wore belts. She had been a secretary before she retired, handling carbon paper over many years, and remembered being caught in the rain several times on the way to work and encountering difficulty removing the black dye from her tights and feet.

Jean's feet had the remnants of blisters to both heels and many of her toes, apparently caused by wearing new black leather shoes on a recent holiday to Madeira where she had done a lot of walking and hadn't worn any tights. On one occasion the walk had caused blisters which had burst, thereby removing any barrier that the skin could provide in preventing the dye from entering her system. This was the source of the black dye that had been identified in her body.

Although the initial complaint was Jean's bowel problem, there was concern that the dye was interfering with her breathing too, as the mediastinal plexus had a low reading. Jean did in fact feel that her breathing was labored. She belonged to a choral society and had found recently that it was difficult to take deep breaths. Thinking she was fighting off some sort of virus she had missed her last two meetings.

The mediastinal plexus

With breathing problems, either the bronchial or mediastinal plexuses are often disturbed by very congested lymphatics nearby. The anterior mediastinum contains many lymph nodes that, if congested, will interfere with the supply of energy to the mediastinum (the space between the lungs). The mediastinum contains the heart, trachea, esophagus, thymus gland, the major blood vessels entering and leaving the heart, lymphatic vessels and nerves (including the vagus and phrenic nerves).

Jean's acupuncture readings for this point, although abnormal, were not very low, but the variety of symptoms associated with disturbance to this plexus can be quite confusing and disabling. If a malfunctioning plexus is not identified due to either congested lymph nodes or lymphatics nearby then no amount of investigations into the associated symptoms will be conclusive. The practitioner is usually left with little alternative to prescriptive drugs to ease the symptoms. Exercise 2 (lungs and upper abdomen; see Appendix 1) is very good for inducing lymphatic drainage of the mediastinal plexus and is effective in restoring the correct communication between the plexus and tissues.

The mesenteric, hypogastric and celiac plexuses are all discussed in Chapter 6. As explained there, many ganglia and plexuses have dual roles to play by way of interconnecting energy fields. For this reason, many patients will gain relief from a wide range of symptoms during the course of the treatment sessions, a fact that is an added incentive for those who subscribe to preventive therapy. The exercises used to enhance the electrical output from all of these plexuses are consequently contained in this case study too. The small intestine plays a major role in bowel abnormalities and many other conditions too, particularly if the food-absorbing process is incomplete because of a faulty energy field. Any undigested food will be hurriedly moved into the colon, where it will irritate the wall of the colon and increase bowel peristalsis and possibly the symptoms discussed earlier. Although there are many reasons why the body malfunctions enough for IBS to develop, poor diet, drug/alcohol abuse and surgery are contributing factors. A low-energy output from one of these nerve plexuses will, without doubt, be instrumental in the condition. Abdominal massage is very effective in restoring energy transmission in the abdominal cavity and subsequently is beneficial in treating IBS. The activity between biological energy fields in the abdominal region is such that this simple massage will often restore energy to many areas of the body. This is another reminder of why the body should be looked upon as a whole unit of interconnecting energy fields, and not sectioned into fragmented sections for diagnosis.

Treatment

It is extremely important that, whenever possible, a partnership between patient and therapist over exercise techniques should be established. This particular method of lymphatic drainage requires the integration that is outlined in the case studies to achieve maximum results. This case study particularly expresses the need for patient participation.

Full details of how to perform the exercises in the following list can be found in Appendix 1.

1. **Reflexology.** To the liver, kidneys, spleen, lungs and subclavian lymph drainage points followed by the large and small intestine, pancreas, lymph cistern, lungs, bladder and womb (see Fig. 7.2, pp 54–55). Massage above and below the clavicles.

2. **Exercise 1, lymph cistern.**

3. **Exercise 2, lungs and upper abdomen.** This exercise clears the lungs and upper abdomen. (Caution: if there is a problem with brittle bones the patient must not put pressure on the ribs, but direct the breath towards the hands.)

4. **Foot rotation.** This exercise stimulates the muscles of the thigh and activates the nerves, which supply energy to the muscles and ligaments of the pelvis. This helps to release any constraint to the sciatic nerve and, combined with Exercise 3 (inguinal drain), is very successful for pelvic and lower back conditions.

5. **Exercise 3, inguinal drain.** This exercise clears the lymphatics of the small intestine, colon and the area around the rectum.

6. **Repeat Exercise 1, lymph cistern.**

7. **Abdominal massage.** An oil which consisted of a base of 10 ml almond, 2 drops camomile with 3 drops of lavender essential oils was tested for its suitability using ISR prior to massage. This is an excellent facility for accurately assessing the patient's acceptance of an oil, particularly in view of nut allergy.

8. **Do-in.** Tap gently either side of the sternum.

9. **Reflexology.** To the liver, kidneys, spleen, lungs, lymph drainage points, large and small intestine, pancreas, lymph cistern, bladder and womb (see Fig. 7.2, pp 54–55).

It would be advisable for the patient to repeat the program once a day for 2 weeks followed by alternate days until symptoms subside.[1] Thereafter, once or twice a week as a lymphatic maintenance regime.

Jean must remove all black leather items from her wardrobe until all of her symptoms have subsided. Black leather can be reintroduced only if the body will accept it and must be rechecked at intervals using ISR.

Patient guide

1. Water: plenty of water is advisable for bowel problems, including diarrhea. Drink at least eight glasses a day.

---

[1] Appendix 2 contains instructions to the patient on how to perform the exercises in Appendix 1.

2. Honey: one teaspoon of honey dissolved in cooled boiled water makes a soothing drink that settles the intestines and also the stomach. Two glasses a day can be a substitute for plain water.

3. If food sensitivities have not been identified it could be beneficial for patients with IBS to avoid the proprietary brands of breakfast cereal that are advertised to keep you 'regular'. They might actually irritate the colon and make the condition worse. If wheat is not suspected as a potential allergen then Weetabix™ for breakfast is very good for constipation. However, ISR should be mastered where possible, as explained earlier, to dispel the uncertainty over foods.

4. Arrowroot: take a quarter of a teaspoon in a drop of warm water each morning to bind the stool. This is extremely beneficial when suffering from diarrhea. Arrowroot can be obtained from most chemists.

5. Miso: it is advisable to take a small amount (equivalent to the small finger nail) each day, half an hour before breakfast and last thing at night (Note: miso should *not* be taken with a hot drink).

Miso is a beneficial addition to the diet for patients suffering from any bowel abnormality. A 1-year-old child attended the clinic with constant loose stools. He had been in and out of hospital and been fully investigated but the doctors could find nothing wrong. Within four days of the child taking a small amount of miso each morning and evening the stools were normal.

Miso is fermented, unpasteurized soya pulp and can be found in some major supermarkets (although care should be taken that it is macrobiotic – see Appendix 3 for suppliers). It contains large amounts of the healthy bacteria *Lactobacillus acidophilus*. In a healthy person, this friendly bacteria is naturally present in the intestines, where it destroys unhealthy bacteria. Unfortunately, antibiotics can destroy the whole colony of healthy bacteria. It is therefore most important to replenish the intestines on a regular basis, especially after bouts of diarrhea and after taking antibiotics, as this can restore intestinal health.

Dr Phillip Evans believes that the regular consumption of acidophilus culture (in some form) is infinitely more important than most other nutritionists envisage. He suggests that acidophilus should be taken on a daily basis, so that the entire bacterial population of the intestine (80% of the solid material of the stools) become lactic-acid organisms. These organisms live only on milk sugar (lactose) and die within 5 days unless milk in some form, or milk sugar, is supplied to them, but they do destroy the gas-forming, disease and odor-producing bacteria, so are very important to the gut (Rowell).

One would presume, therefore, that to be effective and fostered these friendly bacteria must be fed lactose in some form. However, much of my research has involved patients who had taken antibiotics for a considerable length of time, leading one to presume that the colony of natural flora would undoubtedly be depleted. In all of these patients, milk sensitivity was identified. How can milk-sensitive patients restore the healthy flora to their intestinal tract successfully?

From clinical and personal experience, unpasteurized miso is a natural source of this healthy bacteria. Miso is fermented for 12 to 18 months with strains of lactic bacteria that are carefully cultured, usually in Japan, and have been mindfully passed on for many generations. Miso is very rich in these healthy bacteria, and far more effective than any other natural source, including live yogurt. This must be due to the particular strains of lactic bacteria used and, for whatever reason, miso is very effective and most beneficial without lactose. Therefore, replacing the healthy bacteria with miso each day, not only helps to promote healthy intestines but also helps eliminate milk intolerance.

6. Nettle tea: take two cups per day. This tea is excellent for helping to cleanse the system. However, the suitability of this tea for each patient should be checked, as anyone who suffers from high blood pressure could see a rise in pressure if too much is drunk. Care must be taken when prescribing nettle tea.

7. Homeopathic remedies: rhus tox and chamomilla. Many patients have spoken favorably about the effects of these.

8. Oils: ginger, rosemary and peppermint in a base of almond oil have also been successful in

many cases of IBS. Do not exceed the five drops of essential oil to a base oil of 10 ml. To be used for abdominal massage.

Jean responded very quickly to the treatments, once all the offending substances were removed, and she became proficient in all of the exercises. However, she returned a few times each year for a check-up.

AN UNEXPECTED BREAST ABNORMALITY

On one such occasion a lump was discovered in the region of the left breast through reflexology. When this situation presents it should be explained to the patient that it is probably a harmless congested lymph node, and she should be encouraged to check the breast herself. Using the breast zone of the foot in relation to the actual breast, the patient can be directed to where the lump is thought to be. Often, there is no evidence of any lump in the actual breast and the patient should consult her doctor. However, quite remarkably, Jean had attended a mobile unit for a mammogram a few days previously and felt it wiser therefore to wait for the results of this mammogram before bothering her doctor. In the meantime, she was given a reflexology chart for the relevant zones and asked to massage those areas marked on the chart each evening.

The following morning Jean phoned the clinic distraught to say she had received a letter asking her to attend her local hospital to discuss the results of her mammogram.

When Jean attended the hospital, it was confirmed that the mammogram had shown an abnormality. Jean asked if it was her left breast; a surprised doctor replied that it was, and asked if she had suffered any discomfort. Jean explained about the treatment and reflexology at which point the doctor asked if she could examine Jean once more, after which she was asked to have another mammogram.

After this second mammogram Jean was immediately taken into the doctor's room to be told, much to her relief, that her mammogram was clear. The follow-up examination and further mammogram were also clear.

Prior to reflexology, the acupoints for the mammary glands had identified aluminum from antiperspirants. Antiperspirants frequently affect the breasts by blocking their lymphatic drainage. Chemicals can also be absorbed from the small intestine up into the breast because the stomach meridian passes through the breast and a secondary line of the meridian passes along the medial side of each breast. This is how many metals and chemicals get into breast milk and affect the nursing baby (Fox, unpublished work, 1989).

All lumps within the breast tissue should be investigated medically as a first priority.

If breast lumps are being investigated medically, it is advisable that the treatment program be reflexology only, and this for 20 minutes daily.

To help keep the lymphatics of the breast area clear, the following massage and lymph drainage exercises are recommended.

1. **Reflexology.** This should be given for 3 weeks; 10 minutes on each foot for three nights per week will suffice. The routine should always begin and end with the filters (the liver, kidneys, spleen, lungs and lymph drainage points), as well as massage above and below the clavicles.

The following exercises should be completed by the patient once a week in the bath (as long as the patient is tall enough for the toes to touch the end of the bath, otherwise the patient will disappear under the water, like one lady did!). If possible, a bath pillow should be used so that the patient can lie back and relax in the warm water.

1. **Exercise 1, the lymph cistern:** place both hands over the abdomen by the navel and push out the abdomen against your hands without breathing in. Then breathe in while maintaining the pressure and even increasing it for a short time before relaxing and exhaling. Repeat three times. Using a chemical-free baby soap, work up a good lather on your hands before you start the massage. This, combined with the warm water and

the position of the breasts as you lie back in the bath, will prevent any trauma to the breast tissue.

2. **The axillary nodes (armpits):** with plenty of soapsuds on your right hand, massage from the left armpit as far as the clavicle (collarbone), both above and below, thus into the lymph drainage point. Repeat about ten times. Then, with the left hand, massage from the right armpit to the lymph drainage point above and below the right collarbone. See Fig. 7.1b, c (p 52).

3. **Breast drainage:** determine the direction of lymphatic drainage by imagining the face of a clock directly over each breast (see Fig. 7.1a).

In the right breast, the section 11:00 to 1:00 drains directly upwards through nodes into the lymph drainage point behind the right clavicle at the base of the neck. The section 1:00 to 5:00 drains into the nodes behind the intercostal spaces next to the sternum. The section 5:00 to 7:00 drains down into the nodes above the edge of the rib cage (these nodes also drain the lung). The section 7:00 to 11:00 drains outwards and upwards into the axillary nodes of the armpit.

In the left breast, the section 11:00 to 1:00 drains directly upwards through nodes into the lymph drainage point behind the left clavicle at the base of the neck. The section 1:00 to 5:00 drains outwards and then upwards into the axillary nodes. The section 5:00 to 7:00 drains down into the nodes above the edge of the rib cage. The section 7:00 to 11:00 drains inwards to the nodes behind the intercostal spaces next to the sternum.

(i) Using the arrows as a guide, massage each breast, as outlined in Fig. 7.1a.

(ii) Using two or three fingers, massage each space between the ribs either side of the breastbone. Begin just under the collarbone and work in a downwards direction towards the bottom of the breastbone, then work upwards several times. Fig. 7.1d (p 52) shows the position of the lymph nodes between these spaces.

(iii) Then, with the thumb, massage the space just above the edge of the rib cage, from the breastbone, round to the waist area on both sides.

(iv) Hook the fingers just under the ribs on the right side and push out the abdomen for about 5 seconds, repeat once more and then do exactly the same on the left side.

(v) Repeat Exercise 1 (lymph cistern).

(vi) Do-in across the whole chest area.

Although this sounds complicated, it is quite straightforward once you have been through the sequence a few times.

4. **Reflexology.** to the liver, kidneys, spleen, lungs, lymph drainage points, breast, thyroid, ovaries, bladder and womb (see Fig. 7.2, pp 54–55). It is wise to practise reflexology on these extra zones because of the part they play in the endocrine system. Massage above and below the clavicles.

There is a special point at the side of the knee for the breast area (St 36). Sit in a chair, place the palm of the right hand over the right kneecap, encasing the patella (the kneecap). With the fingers spread out, your little finger should just sit in a hollow on the outside of the knee. Massage in this hollow for the right breast. Repeat on the left leg for the left breast. Massage should continue until all tenderness has subsided. This can be performed at any time of the day in the knowledge that the health of the breasts is being maintained.

Supplements that many women have found helpful when suffering from inflammation of the breast area, without any known cause other than premenstrual are:

- evening primrose oil, 1500 mg daily
- magnesium phosphate 4 × 4 daily (tissue salts)
- multivitamin B without yeast
- multivitamin and mineral
- vitamin B6 (check that the dose is not being exceeded with the inclusion of the multivitamin B)
- vitamin E 400 iu daily.

It is important that vitamins and minerals do not contain any artificial colors, flavors or preservatives. See Appendix 3 for suppliers.

As a homeopathic remedy for tender breasts, bryonia, has been most beneficial for many women.

The above-detailed breast drainage exercises, reflexology and massage techniques should

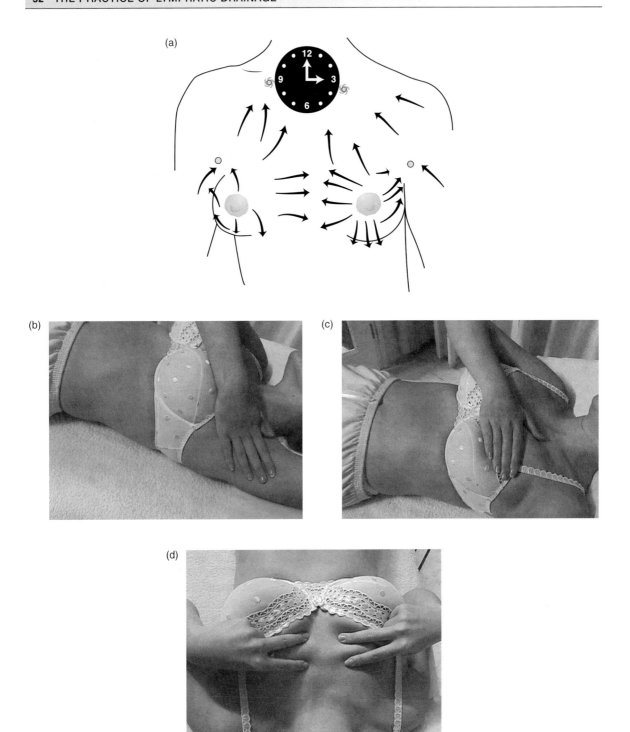

Figure 7.1 Breast drainage exercises.

become part of every woman's breast-care routine and undoubtedly be included in any campaign on breast care. The preventive element of breast lymphatic hygiene must not be overlooked, particularly as our bodies are expected to tolerate inappropriate substances on a daily basis. Harmful chemicals and preservatives in antiperspirants and deodorants should be avoided. If the lymphatic system is functioning normally, the body will not emit body odor. Body odor is a sign that the lymphatic system is congested. Aluminum is just one harmful substance that must be avoided, others still remain unknown for the vast majority of people (see Chapter 15). ISR will provide the means by which every person can assess the suitability of any item of clothing or product for their own body.

The reflexology charts and acupuncture points that are relevant for this case study are shown in Figs 7.2 and 7.3 (pp 54–55) and are to be used in conjunction with ISR and the particular lymphatic drainage techniques that are explained in the text. All of the exercise programs were initially checked against malfunctioning nerve plexuses, ganglia, and congested lymphatic and organs for their improvement value using EAV. The exercises, done correctly, all activated an improvement in nervous energy of the plexi, lymphatics and organs mentioned in this chapter. Practising lymphatic hygiene in this way will protect the body from chemical interactions and congestion.

REFERENCE

Rowell D What *Acidophilus* does. Felmore Health Publications: number 31

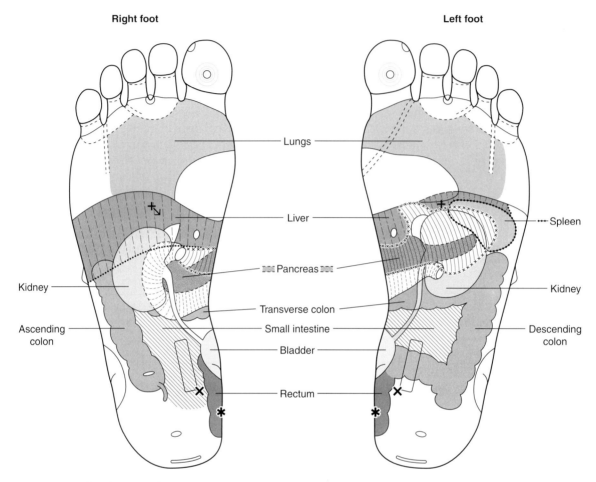

Right foot

Left foot

Lungs

Liver

Spleen

Pancreas

Kidney

Kidney

Transverse colon

Ascending colon

Small intestine

Descending colon

Bladder

Rectum

Figure 7.2 Reflexology chart for the liver, kidneys, spleen, lungs, subclavian lymph drainage points, large and small intestines, pancreas, lymph cistern, bladder, breast, thyroid, ovaries and womb. © F. Fox, used with permission.

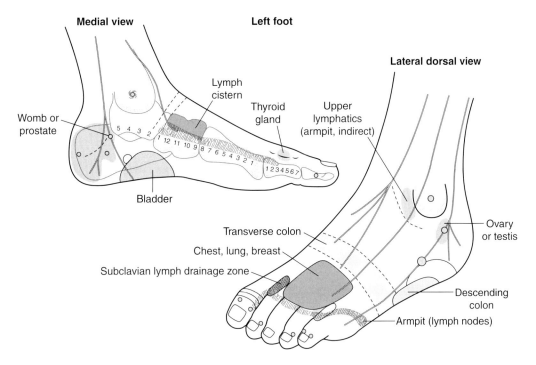

Figure 7.2 (*continued*). Unless otherwise stated, all reflex zones apply to both feet.

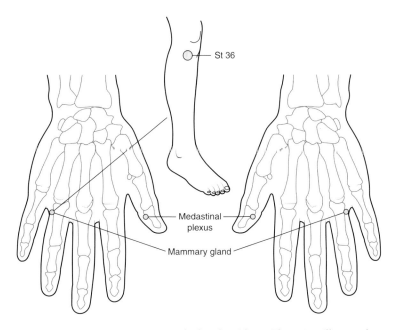

Figure 7.3 Acupuncture points on the hand and knee. The points illustrated are for fingertip testing, assessment, and acupressure only.

8

Arthritis

FIRST VISIT

Peter, a man in his late 50s, walked with great difficulty when he entered the clinic with his wife. His knees were extremely painful and his doctor had diagnosed arthritis.

Arthritis, a condition well known by most people, is an inflammation of any joint. There are more than 100 different types of arthritis and medical classification is based on the cause and progress of the condition. Causes vary, but often infection, metabolic disorders, trauma and immune disorders are listed among its origins. It is generally referred to as wear and tear of the joints but can vary quite considerably from a mild ache and stiffness to very severe pain and possibly, joint deformity.

Osteoarthritis (OA), the most common type of arthritis, is often considered to be an inevitable disease of old age. It can strike after injury but is mainly confined to weight-bearing joints like the knees and hip, and also to the spine. A smooth layer of shiny cartilage covers a normal healthy joint such as the hip or knee. A symptom of the aging process, cartilage deterioration, results in uneven wear and tear on the bone and it is this that causes the pain and stiffness of the joints. Stiffness tends to follow periods of inactivity such as sleeping or sitting, but pain increases at night and often more so in humid weather. Conventional treatment with anti-inflammatory drugs often produces a good reduction in pain level, but little improvement in the arthritic process itself.

Rheumatoid arthritis (RA) is the most severe type of inflammatory joint disease. It is thought to be an autoimmune disorder in which the body produces abnormal antibodies against its own cells and tissues, which damages joints and surrounding soft tissues. Many joints, most commonly those in the hands, wrists, arms, elbows, knees and ankles, become extremely painful, stiff and deformed. In severe cases, there can be considerable destruction of joints: after the inner lining of the joint becomes scarred, scar tissue fills the space within the joint, deforming the underlying bony surfaces and wasting the muscles. Other tissues, including skin, lymph nodes, lungs, the heart, and even the liver and kidneys can be affected by the rheumatoid process (Davies & Stewart 1987). It is, however, a young person's disease, which strikes victims (most of whom are women) between the ages of 20 and 40. People with classic RA have a protein, rheumatoid factor, in their blood and the synovial fluid and associated connective tissue cells proliferate forming a pannus, causing the joint capsule to thicken. This destroys the articular cartilage and in advanced conditions opposing joint surfaces often fuse (Seeley et al 1995).

Conventional treatment attempts to alleviate symptoms and to stop the disease from causing permanent joint destruction. Steroidal anti-inflammatory drugs, gold and even immunosuppressants (particularly those used during transplant operations) are used to prevent whatever autoimmune destruction is going on. But it does appear to be a hit and miss affair in every case and that medication appears only to alleviate the pain (BMA 1990, Heimlich 1990).

Peter, who found that the pain did in fact ease when he continually took his medication, complained that the condition itself hadn't improved.

Peter had some difficulty settling himself onto the treatment couch. On examination the knee joints were badly swollen with limited movement.

His hands too showed signs of the disease. Many of his fingers were swollen, hot and very painful. In particular, the muscles and tendons of his right hand and arm showed signs of tissue change and, upon examination of the axillary glands, painful nodules were obvious.

ISR testing was enlightening. Chlorine was identified in the acupuncture points of the cervical ganglia and also of the small and large intestines, the thoracic aortic plexus, the pancreas and the kidneys.

It is usually presumed that degenerative diseases, except those that stem from genetic faults, are linked to infection, especially viral infection. However, the origins of degenerative disease are also thought to lie in faulty physiology. Early detection and correction of physiological faults in the body can aid the prevention or recovery from degenerative disease. An appropriate way of correcting any faults that underlie or threaten disease is therefore desirable, and a way does exist.

It is the energy fields in and around the body that can direct the therapist towards these faults as they vibrate with the relevant information. This information must be accessed so that the fault can be corrected otherwise healing will not take place. Correction of energy fields can be achieved in a number of ways: a homeopathic remedy will vibrate an opposing energy to the energy field in question; light will also vibrate energy, so too will acupuncture. However, this is not enough. What is required is the integration of various therapies that will manipulate and harmonize the repair mechanisms of the body to sustain the healing process. The missing link in

many areas of healing, and an important feature in this integrated therapy, is the removal of those substances responsible for the malfunctioning fields. This is achieved by using breathing and massage techniques to encourage the safe removal of the offending substance through lymphatic drainage. Then and only then will energetic interactions of organs and tissues be complete and will we have any chance of stopping degenerative diseases like RA in their tracks.

The calcium deposits that form within joints and are the cause of so much suffering are the end product of faulty metabolism, primarily due to a physiological fault. Therefore the prime objective must be to correct the fault by removing the toxic congestion. This will re-establish the correct energy field and reduce the incidence of calcium deposits forming. Early detection of a malfunctioning energy field is, of course, the key to effective prevention of disease by enabling the body to recover quickly from the initial stages of disease with minimal damage giving a better chance of recovery.

The word 'toxins' is used as a broad term throughout this book to describe any substance whose magnetic field is so out of harmony with the biomagnetic patterns of the human body that it actually interferes with physiological functions, especially when present in significant levels. Such substances come from many sources, but it was very obvious where Peter's were coming from. The smell of soap powder from his clothes was overpowering – this was an obvious case of chemical overload, particularly of chlorine.

Chlorine is found as salt in foods, as a condiment and as a preservative, especially in processed foods. It is also present in the public water supply, washing powders and washing liquids, drugs (antibacterial, analgesic and anesthetic), wood preservative, contaminated fruit and vegetables (which absorb chemicals more rapidly), bleach, some denture cleaners and swimming pools.

Chlorine, like any other substance lodged in the lymphatics in significant quantity, can distort vital nerve impulses. The following nerve stations were not emitting the correct frequency to sustain normal body functions and Peter's symptoms were proof of this breakdown:

- the cervical ganglia
- the thoracic aortic plexus.

Cervical ganglia

The three pairs of cervical ganglia lie immediately in front of the cervical vertebrae in the middle and lower parts of the neck and sit between the carotid artery and the jugular vein (see Fig. 5.2, p 27). Collectively, they supply nerve signals to the thyroid, parathyroid and thymus glands. A malfunction of these ganglia disturbs the balanced production of thyroxine, calcitonin and parathormone; the two latter hormones control the level of calcium in the blood. When they are in balance, calcium metabolism in the body is normal. However, if there is an imbalance then calcium is wasted through the liver, passing through the bile ducts into the duodenum. The initial bile ducts can be blocked with calcium and gallstones can form in the gall bladder. Calcium spurs and deposits are another indication that calcium is not being used by the body efficiently. Deposits of calcium can form wherever the circulation of blood is reduced due to spasm, pressure or injury. This is why many past injuries succumb to arthritis in later life and why, after a bone has been broken, the formation of calcium can be seen on X-ray at the site of the break, making that part of the bone stronger. When the levels of calcium in the body are too low, white flecks appear in the fingernails, and cramps can occur. The vagus nerve, which is involved with heart and lung function, passes through the neck close to the cervical ganglia, so any congestion here can quickly affect these organs too.

Rheumatoid arthritis appears to develop from faulty, incomplete nucleoprotein metabolism. Uric acid, the end product of nucleoprotein metabolism, is not converted into urea and various urates as efficiently as it should. As a result, uric acid builds up in connective tissue, especially where there is poor circulation due

to injury or loss of energy, as a result of a congested lymph node, nerve supply or a malfunctioning organ. Excessive uric acid can also build up in the bloodstream if the kidneys cannot handle it. This can cause deposits of uric acid to crystallize and trigger a protective response from the immune system, which causes inflammation and pain.

Thoracic aortic plexus

The thoracic aortic plexus, situated on the aorta just below the base of the heart, is responsible for the blood supply to that part of the pancreas that controls nucleoprotein metabolism and therefore uric acid production. Usually, when the thoracic aortic plexus is burdened, a spasm will form in the thoracic spine, in particular T2 and T3, which should respond to massage once the plexus has recovered.

Explaining the source of the problem

It was explained to Peter and his wife that, when too much soap powder is used in a washing machine, the rinse cycle is unable to remove the excess residue and a considerable amount remains on the clothes. If this is repeated on each wash, then the amount of chlorine left on the clothes builds up. The skin, being very porous, absorbs these chemicals, both from the clothes worn during the day and also from the bedclothes. Not only can this be harmful, but it does very little for the cleanliness of the clothes and further pollutes the environment. Although the chloride ion (Cl^-) is vital to nerve function, in excess it is dangerous.

Unfortunately, Peter's wife reacted badly to this information. She assumed total responsibility for her husband's problem because she used too much soap powder in the washing machine. Taken aback, she questioned why she too wasn't suffering from arthritis, as all the washing was done together. This is fair comment. However, it is due in the main to the individual make-up of the person involved. Although individuals inherit various features, including immunity, from their ancestors, they remain unique and, for this reason, will react independently to any substance. This fact is recognized and used to advantage by the ISR, which directs the therapist towards the relevant integrated therapy specifically for that patient. This recognition should also be applied to medication – what is appropriate for one person's set of symptoms is not necessarily correct for another.

Opinion is divided as to what actually causes arthritis: chronic infection, a hereditary factor or a malfunction of the immune system. In the Western world millions of pounds are spent each year on drugs and joint replacement operations but the fact remains that medicine is at a loss as to the cause of its dominance. Without question, the immune system will be defective and the reason for this will be a congested lymphatic system. For many sufferers, though, there is a simple solution: find the underlying cause of the physiological fault. This will prevent unnecessary drug pollution of the body, less congestion of the lymphatic system and a saving of millions of pounds for a struggling health service. Arthritis and rheumatic diseases in general constitute the major cause of chronic disability in the United States. It is estimated that 16 million persons suffer from a crippling disease that they call arthritis and which is severe enough to interfere with their activities of daily living (O'Toole 1997).

Treatment and contraindications

Lymphatic congestion rarely happens overnight and by the time inflammation and pain are a part of the arthritic's life the degenerative process will have been established. For this reason the therapist will have to decide how much treatment should be given on any one occasion. This can be assessed by way of ISR and the acupuncture points for each patient. The exercise program accompanying this case study is designed to clear lymphatic congestion and therefore the patient's filters should be sufficiently energized to deal with the onslaught of toxins effectively. This cannot be achieved by

rushing through the program because the exercises look straightforward. They *are* simple exercises but they are very effective in stimulating lymphatic flow and should not be underestimated. It would not be sensible to encourage a stagnant lymphatic system to flow all at once on a first treatment. It might be prudent in certain circumstances (Chapter 11 explains this effectively) to use only reflexology for the first treatment, giving the patient the reflex zones to work on at home. This will reduce the likelihood of a reaction and will allow the body to adapt to the cleansing process. During a flare-up of symptoms, which will undoubtedly result in inflammation, reflexology is a useful tool and will bring about good results.

With the exception of certain massage techniques that the professional therapist is familiar with, the following treatment program is easy for any arthritic to follow at home, but guidance should be given by the therapist. It might be practical to introduce a new step every 2 weeks, provided that the continuity of reflexology is maintained and is your final step in each treatment session.

Full details of how to perform the exercises in the following list can be found in Appendix 1.

1. **Reflexology.** To the liver, kidney, spleen, lungs and subclavian lymph drainage points, and massage above and below the clavicles (see Fig. 8.1, pp 66–67).
2. **Exercise 1, the lymph cistern.**
3. **The red light massage.** This exercise clears the cervical lymph nodes, permitting the cervical ganglia to function to their optimum ability. It is so called because massaging the sides of the neck can easily be done while sitting at traffic lights. As the thyroid and parathyroid glands are dependent upon nerve impulses from the cervical ganglia, it would be most beneficial for this exercise to become a daily activity for the prevention of other conditions, for instance, hypothyroidism (which causes tiredness and can contribute to obesity), hyperthyroidism

(which can lead to weight loss) and osteoarthritis and osteoporosis (which are due to faulty calcium metabolism) can all benefit from this massage. As the heart and lungs can also benefit from the energetic interaction that is encouraged by this massage, it can pay dividends to be rigorous in its application. It will, however, take about 3 weeks for the nerve impulses from the ganglia to return to normal.

4. **Massage to both legs.** Muscles should be soft and supple. However, in the arthritic patient this is seldom the case. In severe cases muscles become dry, tough and hard, as the muscle fibers stick together and can't be separated. This is due to lymphatic and vascular congestion, in which the muscles become sealed off from their supply of lymph and blood. When fresh oxygenated aterial blood is prevented from nourishing the muscles they start to degenerate, lose their elasticity and become inflexible. Lymph normally provides the lubrication that is essential if muscle fusion is to be prevented. Unfortunately, when lymph is in short supply there is friction and those muscles that are usually able to move freely and separately will eventually coalesce. Muscles that are strangled in this way cannot hope to move a joint. Inflammation and pain will eventually occur as a result of the muscles pulling on joint tissues and massage is needed in all cases of arthritis to get the circulation of lymph and blood back into the degenerated muscles. After years of being starved of vital nourishment and electrical stimuli in this way, re-establishing circulation to the hard fibrous muscles that are seen in many cases of arthritis will require considerable time and attention. It will be worth the effort and often the results will be felt immediately. Increasing the volume of lymph offers maximum energy to the cells and only sufficient volume will ensure cell normality. Therefore, once the physiological faults have been corrected, enabling proper transmission of energy to organs and tissues, deep muscle massage will help to restore the volume of lymph to these struggling muscles. Muscles lying against the bone will usually be the ones that are tight, hard and the most painful, but massaging across the fibers in a deep slow

motion will bring about renewed circulation that is so necessary for muscle flexibility and therefore reduced pain.

Providing the legs are free from inflammation, the patient might want to massage his or her own legs.

Uric acid crystals and waste from the tissues will eventually be removed by the liver, kidneys, spleen and lungs following massage to the affected limbs, for this reason, reflexology to the corresponding areas for the filters must follow any massage.

5. **Reflexology.** To the liver, kidney, spleen, lungs and drainage points. It might be necessary at this point to assess the acupuncture points for the liver, kidney, spleen and lungs using ISR. If a spasm forms, suggesting they are low in energy, ISR can determine the requirement of a homeopathic remedy in support of the filters as the system clears. In this instance it would be advisable to see the patient again after 3 weeks to repeat the first three steps of the therapy. However, the efficiency of Peter's filters on this first appointment allowed for Exercise 2 (lungs and upper abdomen) to be included as part of his treatment program.

Second treatment

1. **Reflexology.** To the liver, kidney, spleen, lungs and drainage points (see Fig. 8.1, pp 66–67).
2. **Exercise 1, lymph cistern.**
3. **The red light massage.**
4. **Exercise 2, lungs and upper abdomen.** This exercise clears the lungs and upper abdomen. (Caution: if there is a problem with brittle bones the patient must not put pressure on the ribs, but direct the breath towards the hands.)
5. **Repeat Exercise 1, lymph cistern.** As a reminder for arthritics, the cistern has to be clear to allow vitamin D, which is fat soluble, to be absorbed in the chyme from the intestines. An important vitamin, it is required by the body to regulate the balance of calcium and phosphate; it aids the absorption of calcium from the intestine and is essential for strong bones and teeth. Too much vitamin D is harmful,

can lead to abnormal calcium deposits in the soft tissues and detrimental for people with arthritis, it is still needed by the body. Diet is by far the best way of receiving vitamin D – oily fish (such as sardines, herring, salmon and tuna), liver and egg yolk all contain this vitamin. In the body, vitamin D is formed by the action of ultraviolet rays in sunlight on a specific chemical in the skin. Therefore, if sun doesn't cause a problem, it could be beneficial in small doses.

6. **Abdominal massage.**
7. **Repeat Exercise 1, lymph cistern.**
8. **Do-in.** Gently on the upper part of the sternum and thyroid.
9. **Reflexology.** To the liver, kidneys, spleen, lungs and drainage points followed by the thyroid gland, pituitary gland, adrenal gland, heart, large and small intestines, pancreas, lymph cistern and, in Peter's case, to the knee area (see Fig. 8.1, pp 66–67). The above reflexology points to be done three times a week for a total of 15 minutes.

Peter rang one week later, expressing great sorrow at having to cancel his next appointment. Although the massage had improved mobility of his legs, his wife would not accept the fact that too much soap powder could be a factor in his condition. He could not convince her that the treatment was worth taking a step further to see if there was any long-term relief. As he was not prepared to subject himself to his wife's antagonism, which would cause him more stress, he had decided to withdraw from treatment. He was adamant that he would continue to use his chart for reflexology and would guard against the overuse of chlorine from other sources.

Unfortunately, Peter's case couldn't be concluded successfully. However, Dorothy, a retired shop assistant, was also suffering badly from arthritis of the knees and her case study shows how a positive approach to the therapy stopped the arthritic progress. Lymphatic congestion revealed a similarity to that identified in Peter's condition and describes how Dorothy continued the treatment program

and gained enormous relief from the following steps:

1. **Reflexology.** To the liver, kidneys, spleen, lungs and lymph drainage points.
2. **Exercise 1, lymph cistern.**
3. **The red light massage.**
4. **Exercise 2, lungs and upper abdomen.**
5. **Repeat Exercise 1, lymph cistern.**
6. **Abdominal massage.**
7. **Repeat Exercise 1, lymph cistern.**
8. **Do-in.** as above.
9. **Exercise 4, the four-step.** This helps to correct the nerve supply of the celiac plexus.

The celiac plexus is large and is a direct continuation from the solar plexus. It subdivides into the gastric, hepatic and splenic plexuses and is located on the aorta close to the diaphragm. This is the nerve supply to the pancreas that controls the production of enzymes that manage protein metabolism. Most arthritic sufferers appear to have a problem with this function, resulting in food sensitivity. A spasm can also form in the thoracic spine, usually between T5 and T12, which explains why many patients with multiple food sensitivities complain of pain in this region.

Identification of food sensitivities is very important at this stage. Removing the suspect foodstuff from the diet will reduce the stress this imposes and will encourage the body to heal more rapidly. ISR is fascinating to use for the identification of the offending foods and remarkably accurate.

Food sensitivities

Without exception, patients with arthritis are sensitive to certain foods, the main culprit being milk and products made from milk. However, many patients feel uncomfortable with the idea that milk should be eliminated from their diet, as most people believe that milk and its by-products are our only source of calcium. Annemarie Colbin is one of America's foremost experts on the relationship between food and health. She writes (Colbin 1990):

The calcium craze not only is unwarranted but may have considerably damaging effects. This is especially true of dairy products, often touted for their calcium content but also very high in protein – one of the major causes of osteoporosis and implicated in many other illnesses. Calcium can be drained by foods that cause an acid condition in the body (protein and carbohydrate-rich foods) and those that draw calcium out of the tissues. These include a high *consumption of protein, salt, caffeine, vinegar, alcohol, and sugar.*

Colbin suggests that the body can get sufficient calcium from leafy greens (especially the kind that are cooked, such as broccoli, which offers the highest ratio of calcium to calories of any food):

Calcium is also present in beans, nuts, seeds (sesame seeds have 10 times the calcium of milk) and especially sea vegetables. For those who are not vegetarians, calcium can be obtained by eating fish with bones (such as canned salmon) or making soup with bones and adding one tablespoon of organic cider vinegar, which releases the calcium and makes it available in the broth. (Colbin 1990)

Although a high consumption of vinegar is detrimental and can drain calcium from bones, a good quality cider vinegar can assist in the removal of calcium from surrounding tissues, which is helpful to arthritics. The dosage is one teaspoon of cider vinegar in a glass of water taken with a meal.

Lack of absorption can be caused by such factors as insufficient phosphorus or magnesium, lack of sunlight or vitamin D. (Colbin 1990)

Or the incorrect electrical communications between plexuses and tissues.

Osteoporosis

Osteoporosis has received increased media attention with the assumption that calcium supplements will prevent this major health problem. Women of all ages are ready to accept that once the menopause is upon them, their bones will start to crumble. Calcium tablets are becoming a part of everyday living not only for postmenopausal women, but also for those in

their 30s, who are hoping that the early intervention will save them from this disease. Unfortunately, when the calcium level in the blood is too high, calcium is wasted through the liver, as it passes with the bile through the bile ducts into the duodenum. The bile ducts may become blocked with calcium and gallstones can form in the gall bladder. It is far more beneficial to ensure that the body is functioning efficiently and is therefore capable of absorbing minerals like calcium naturally than to introduce them artificially. The body has more than enough to contend with without adding unnecessary supplements.

One woman who was suffering from osteoporosis visited the clinic for help in identifying food sensitivities in the hope of improving her condition. Following the exercises outlined for Peter and Dorothy, and eliminating milk and its by-products from her diet, the condition improved and her bone density has increased year on year. This patient also had mercury leaking into her system from a filling (see Chapter 11).

Dr Gwynne Davies, a clinical ecologist, writer and lecturer who suffers from arthritis, has done much research on the subject. In his article entitled *You don't have to live with arthritis* (Davies 1996), he says:

Eating dairy products can increase the rate at which calcium is lost from the bones and so hasten osteoporosis. As well as being high in calcium, dairy products are also high protein foods. If we have too much protein in the diet from milk products or any other source, such as meat, fish, or eggs, the body has to get rid of the excess. To do this the kidneys must lose calcium as they cleanse the blood of excess waste. People in the United States and Scandinavia consume more dairy products than anywhere else in the world, yet they have the highest rate of osteoporosis. Cows milk contains the accumulated pesticides that have been sprayed on to the grain to feed the cattle, and the pastureland, and the female hormones given to cows to increase milk production and body fat. Some milk has also been shown to contain trace metals and radioactivity at levels higher than those permissible in drinking water. Some 20% of milk producing cows in America are infected with leukaemia viruses, which, because the milk is pooled when collected, infects the whole milk supply. These cancer-inducing viruses are resistant to being killed by pasteurisation and have been recovered from the supermarket supplies. Can it really be coincidence that the highest rates of leukemia are found in children aged 3–13 who consume the most milk products, and in dairy farmers who, as a profession have the highest rates of leukemia in any group.

I hope the above text will stem any fears for those who must eliminate milk from their diet to stay healthy, including children who are milk sensitive. Calcium can be obtained from many foods, including almonds, raisins, apricots, prunes, raspberries, dates, dandelion, any greens, rhubarb, beetroot, cress, sesame seeds, spinach and turnip.

Anti-inflammatory drugs

Twenty-seven years ago I was informed by a consultant rheumatologist that my condition (rheumatoid arthritis) was not sufficiently advanced to treat and that it could be managed with painkillers. Thankfully, some years later I identified milk as a sensitive food and eliminated it from my diet, thus avoiding the need for drugs. A patient suffering from the same condition consulted me a few years ago. She was told that anti-inflammatory drugs would control the pain and inflammation but that her condition was also not advanced enough for her doctor to treat it. Treatment usually means surgery and the replacement of the deformed joint. However, help is available before this is necessary, by way of correcting any physiological faults. Although drugs will ease pain, the condition might well be accelerating and the drugs could actually cause further damage to other areas of the body.

Drugs often settle into the very tissues where pain exists, and this is due to the particularly poor circulation in those areas. Recovery can be hindered as the tissues become clogged and attract calcium, causing pain and stiffness in the joint and muscles. The intestines too can suffer, and many arthritics will confirm that the drugs they take make them constipated. Low energy fields in the pelvic organs, resulting in weak muscles, have been identified in people who have taken either sleeping tablets or painkillers

for as little as 3 weeks. The effect this can have on the spine is quite remarkable (see Chapter 6) and skeletal problems can quickly follow, along with more painkillers.

This was exactly what happened to Dorothy. She originally contacted me because her next door neighbor had received help with a back problem and Dorothy had suddenly developed what appeared to be sciatica. Totally disabled by this pain she displayed tremendous courage just coming to the clinic. Remarkably, a cold and flu preparation that she had taken for only 5 nights was identified in the hypogastric plexus. Apparently, many of her joints and muscles had been aching, her knees were particularly painful and she thought she was getting the flu so, to aid sleep and reduce pain, she had taken this preparation. When given the opportunity, the body will heal itself very quickly and the speed with which the sciatica receded was due to the limited time (5 nights) the cold preparation had to suppress nervous energy in the area. Dorothy's abdominal muscles were tight, which is inclined to happen very quickly, causing sciatica and prompting patients to say 'but I only lifted a cup and my back went'. It is not the physical lifting of the cup or any other movement that causes this response, it is the distortion of energy, usually from the hypogastric plexus to the small intestine. This invariably causes a stasis in the small intestine on the corresponding side as the trapped sciatic nerve. If caught immediately, the congested lymph vessels and nodes responsible in the abdomen/pelvis area will have little time to do much damage other than to spasm the muscles. Dorothy was able to benefit from immediate attention and as soon as the muscles in her abdomen became pliable, discharging of the congested lymph through the nodes eased the searing pain. Although she moved gingerly off the treatment couch, she was grinning from ear to ear.

It is important to identify faults as quickly as possible in the hope they can be corrected immediately, reducing the likelihood of further damage. Dorothy became an attentive patient after this episode and, with her cooperation, was able to receive help for her arthritic knees by reducing the amount of soap powder in her washing machine and following the treatment program.

Although Dorothy's doctor had warned her that she would probably need replacement joints at some point, this has not happened. When the muscles of the lower limbs started to respond to massage and became more pliable, the pain to the knees became less severe. This encouraged her to eat sensibly and she was extremely vigilant over her diet. The knee joints have not altered in shape very much but pain has significantly reduced. She walks as much as possible and is now able to enjoy ballroom dancing.

PATIENT GUIDE: TIPS AND SUPPLEMENTS THAT HAVE HELPED ARTHRITIC CONDITIONS

1. The first priority is to reduce the amount of soap powder in the washing machine and to put the machine through a few extra rinse cycles for 2 or 3 weeks. Bicarbonate of soda is the antidote for chlorine (discovered thanks to the Mora machine) and one tablespoon added to the final rinse will help to eliminate and neutralize the magnetic field of the chemicals.

2. Use ISR: check the foods and products that are suitable for your body.

3. Water filter: purchase as soon as possible to remove excess chemicals from your drinking water (*Note*: not all filters remove chlorine).

4. Massage to the affected joints is highly recommended, preferably by a qualified therapist who will be familiar with the procedure for inflammation. If massage is self-administered, do be very careful to make sure that the affected joints are not inflamed before you commence! (Inflamed joints will be red and the temperature of the skin over the joint will be higher than normal.)

5. Epsom Salts: put some in your bath: the sulfur content appears to repel uric acid magnetically. Put one tablespoon into a glass of warm water and place a large cotton handkerchief in the glass and leave for 15 minutes. Squeeze out the excess water and fold the hankie into a square, then place it on the affected joint. The handkerchief must be left on the joint overnight and the treatment should be repeated on three consecutive nights. This can help to remove excess calcium from the joint and is particularly effective for knees.

6. Add one-quarter of a teaspoon of sodium bicarbonate B.P. to a glass of cooled boiled water 1 day a week for 3 weeks: this will help to eliminate chlorine from the body. *Caution*: this must not be undertaken until reflexology to the kidneys, liver, spleen and lungs has been performed for at least 3 weeks. Check first with your GP if you are on a low sodium diet, or if you have high blood pressure, heart, kidney or liver problems, as the balance of sodium/potassium levels will be significant to you.

7. Magnesium: appears to repel calcium in the tissues, so is beneficial as a first (not long-term) measure towards clearing out calcium formation. It is thought that calcium cannot be absorbed by the body without sufficient magnesium (Pitchford 1993).

8. New Era Tissue Salts magnesium phosphate (no. 8) and calcium fluoride (no. 1): are part of homeopathy and are taken together for inflammation and to relieve pain. These can be obtained from most large chemists and health stores. These remedies, like any other, can be checked for their effectiveness through ISR.

9. Selenium: is needed as an anti-inflammation agent. Arthritis sufferers are often lacking in this supplement. It is likely to be missing from the diet because of the low levels in the soil in the UK. Studies show that heart disease, cancer and degenerative disorders are more prevalent when selenium is absent in the diet. The richest sources are seafoods, grains and plants, but obviously these are dependent upon the soil content.

10. Vitamin C: 2 g a day for the relief of pain.

11. Vitamin E: 400–600 iu per day helps the circulation.

12. Extra virgin olive oil: one teaspoon half-hour before breakfast each morning appears to oil the joints and thereby give greater mobility, with an added bonus of ease of bowel movements. I have had rave reports from arthritics about this.

13. Halibut oil: one capsule each day for its vitamin D content.

14. Aspirin: *Note*: aspirin stimulates the adrenal gland and can cause damage if taken in large doses over long periods. One of the main medical first aids against osteoarthritis.

15. Arnica: this homeopathic remedy stimulates the adrenal glands and also soothes the tension in the body that is caused by arthritis.

16. Exercise: too much can be counterproductive – little and often is by far the best policy.

17. Miso: twice a day.

18. Water: drink eight glasses of water a day for 3 days, do this for 3 weeks if treating yourself.

19. Hydrogen peroxide (H_2O_2) 3% food grade: use as an alternative to chlorine. It counteracts unwanted bacterial invaders. Add 8 oz of 3% H_2O_2 to your wash in place of bleaches with fumes. Add $\frac{1}{4}$ cup to a sink full of cold water to soak light vegetables, i.e. lettuce, for 20 minutes.

Add 8 oz of white sugar and 4–8 oz H_2O_2 in 1 gallon of water and use as an insecticide spray.

Add 2 oz H_2O_2 to your regular washing formula in the dishwasher; your glasses will sparkle.

GALLSTONES

One of the causes of misdirected calcium in the body due to a malfunction in the nerve supply can be gallstones.

The simple elimination of gallstones

The principal disorder of the gallbladder, with which most other problems are associated, is the formation of gallstones. Gallstones are composed of either cholesterol or bile pigments and calcium compounds. Symptoms occur when a gallstone gets stuck in the duct leading from the gallbladder. This causes intense pain in the upper right side of the abdomen or between the shoulder blades, and might make the sufferer feel sick and possibly vomit. Indigestion made worse by fatty foods often seems to be associated with gallstones, flatulence too. X-ray or ultrasound scans of the gallbladder are performed to identify the presence of gallstones. In some cases, drug treatment can be used especially if the stones are small and do not contain calcium, but surgical removal of the gallbladder is carried out in 95% of cases.

If you want to avoid drugs or the surgeon's knife, here is a simple, painless and quick way of eliminating the stones (Dulwich Health Society 1997):

Drink 2 litres of pure apple juice for 6 days. On the sixth day, skip dinner. At 9 pm, take one or two tablespoons of Epsom salts dissolved in a little warm water. At 10 pm, shake together 4 oz unrefined cold-pressed olive oil and 2 oz lemon juice and drink. Go to bed immediately and lie on your right side with your right knee drawn up towards your chin. Remain in this position for 30 minutes before going to sleep. Prepare another Epsom salts solution in case you need it in the middle of the night. The next morning, you should pass stones that are as soft as putty.

The reflexology charts and acupuncture points that are relevant for this case study are shown in Figs 8.1 and 8.2 (pp 66–68) and are to be used in conjunction with ISR and lymphatic drainage techniques. Practising lymphatic hygiene in this way will protect you from the hazards of chemical interactions and congestion.

REFERENCES

British Medical Association 1990 Complete family encyclopedia. Dorling Kindersley, London, p 131
Colbin A 1990 Calcium crazy. What Doctors Don't Tell You; 1(6)
Davies G 1996 You don't have to live with arthritis. Allergy newsletter, number 56, spring issue
Davies S, Stewart A 1987 Nutritional medicine. Pan Books, London, p 257
Dulwich Health Society 1997 Failsafe apple juice and oil flush (letter to the editor). What Doctors Don't Tell You; 7(11)
Heimlich J 1990 What your doctor won't tell you. HarperPerennial, New York
Oschman J 2000 Energy medicine. Harcourt Publishers, London
O'Toole M T (ed) 1997 Miller–Keane encyclopedia and dictionary of medicine, nursing and allied health, 6th edn. W B Saunders, Philadelphia, p 127
Pitchford P 1993 Healing with whole food. North Atlantic Books, Berkeley, California, p 178
Seeley R R, Stephens T D, Tate D A 1995 Anatomy and physiology, 3rd edn. CV Mosby, St Louis, p 256

FURTHER READING

Colbin A 1998 Food and our bones: the natural way to prevent osteoporosis. Plume Books, New York
Oschman J 2000 Energy medicine. Harcourt Publishers, London
Pitchford P 1993 Healing with whole food. North Atlantic Books, Berkeley, California
Randolph T G, Moss R W 1984 Allergies. Thorsons, Northampton
Stein M 2000 Vinegar. Nature's secret weapon. The Windsor Group, Chelmsford, Essex

USEFUL ADDRESSES

Action Against Allergy
PO Box 278, Twickenham, Middlesex TW1 4QQ
Tel: 020 8892 2111

The Arthritis Association
First Floor Suite, 2 Hyde Gardens, Eastbourne, East Sussex BN21 4PN
Tel: 01323 416550

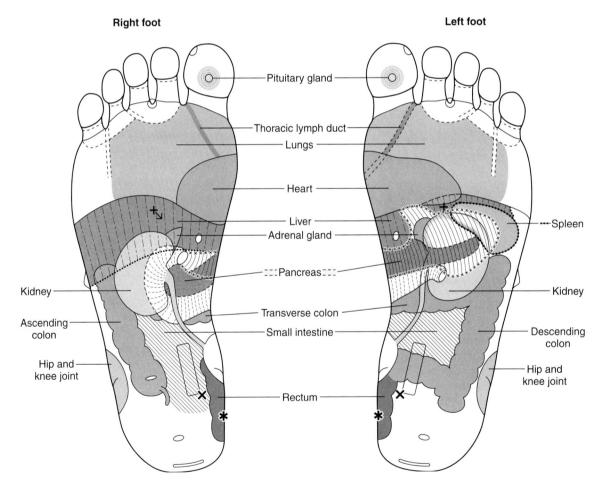

Right foot **Left foot**

Pituitary gland
Thoracic lymph duct
Lungs
Heart
Liver
Adrenal gland
Spleen
Pancreas
Kidney
Kidney
Ascending colon
Transverse colon
Small intestine
Descending colon
Hip and knee joint
Hip and knee joint
Rectum

Figure 8.1 Reflexology chart for the liver, kidneys, spleen, lungs, subclavian lymph drainage points, thyroid gland, pituitary gland, adrenal gland, heart, large and small intestines, pancreas, lymph cistern and knee. © F. Fox, used with permission.

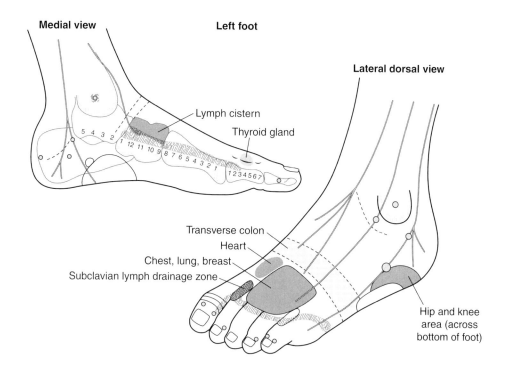

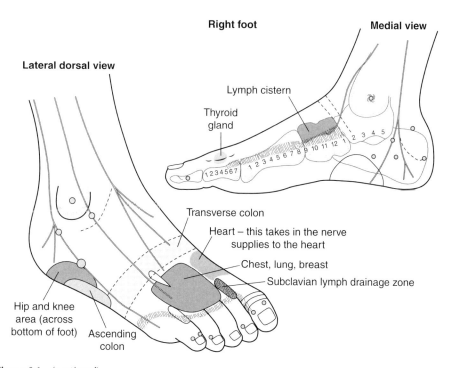

Figure 8.1 (*continued*).

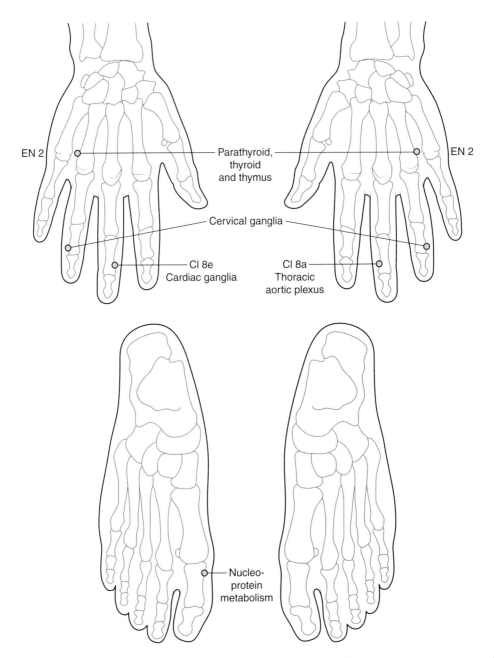

Figure 8.2 Relevant acupuncture points. The points illustrated are for fingertip testing, assessment, and acupressure only.

9

Degeneration of the cervical spine

FIRST VISIT

Elaine was 43 and a hairdresser. She complained of pain in the cervical and thoracic areas of the spine; this was causing a great deal of discomfort, especially while she was working. The pain made her weary, bad tempered and unable to sleep at night. After trying different pillows, a neck collar and sleeping tablets, which made her very drowsy during the day, she was becoming distraught. Her husband was complaining too, her restlessness during the night was disturbing his sleep. Moving into a spare room had not gone down too well; he felt rejected. Her 20-year-old son, she suspected, was taking drugs; he would arrive home from a night out, drenched in sweat. As his relationship with his father was not good at the best of times, she was shouldering this responsibility alone. Most conversations undertaken in the home ended in conflict and consequently any discussion with her husband concerning her son was totally out of the question. Work being her only means of escape, she needed to continue.

A hospital consultation had revealed cervical degeneration of the spine due to arthritis. She was told she had to live with the condition. Medication consisted of anti-inflammatory drugs and painkillers. Although her pain had eased, stiffness and movement were a problem. EAV and ISR testing indicated congestion of the lymphatics of the small intestine, with further low energy readings for the ovaries, thyroid, pituitary, duodenum, jejunum and cervical ganglia.

As explained in Chapter 8, the cervical ganglia sit between the carotid artery and the jugular vein, at the sides of the neck. One of their functions is to supply the nerve signals to the thyroid and parathyroid glands to balance the production of calcitonin and parathormone, the hormones that control the level of calcium in the blood. Any distortion of these nerve signals will disrupt the mechanism of these very important glands, resulting in faulty calcium absorption and could very well lead to osteoarthritis or osteoporosis. If blood levels of calcium are too high, then deposits of calcium can form wherever there is reduced circulation of blood. If they are too low, then the bones will suffer. The external branches of the cervical ganglia are numerous and communicate with many other nerves, including the cranial, thyroid and four upper spinal nerves. Headaches, tiredness, loss of weight and of course pain in the upper spine resulting from arthritis or osteroporosis are just a few of the symptoms that can be experienced with distortion of energy to these ganglia. Any fault relating to the cervical ganglia can easily be detected by testing the conveniently located acupuncture point on the lateral side of the distal joint of the fourth finger of each hand. If, for example, the fault lies with the thyroid or parathyroid glands, respectively, this can be identified long before diseases like osteoarthritis and osteoporosis become clinically diagnosable. Innervation of the organs can be corrected with lymph drainage and the glands tuned without delay to enable the body to recover quickly from the initial stages of disease.

The substances that were responsible for the congestion in Elaine's case study were chlorine and silver. Identifying the source of the offending substances was not too difficult in this instance: Elaine had stopped wearing rubber gloves when she was using hair preparations in her salon. Many of these substances contain chlorine or chloride. Silver was probably being absorbed from her jewelry, in particular the thick chain around her neck, which fell just about where the thyroid gland is situated. The silver chain was removed and the ISR technique was demonstrated to Elaine, showing her the effect the chain was having on her body. The muscle between her finger and thumb became so painful during the test as she held the chain in her left hand that she cried out. Checking the acupuncture point for the thyroid gland without the chain produced a normal reading and no spasm. This evidence indicated that the chain, which included silver as one of its constituents, had a magnetic field that was out of harmony with that of the thyroid gland and was interfering with its nerve supply and function every time it was worn. Other sources of silver include electroplated wrist watches and bands, buckles, earrings, brooches, medals, rings, dental amalgam (fillings usually comprise 40% silver).

Further tests with the chain removed were conducted on acupuncture points that demonstrated low readings when the chain was being worn. Some responded equally, others showed just a slight improvement, this suggested that silver had actually been absorbed into the body in those areas. One such area was the cervical ganglia.

These facts would suggest that silver was antagonistic to Elaine's body, the result of which was a lowering of the electrical output of nervous energy whenever she came into contact with it. For this reason it was suggested that she stop wearing silver jewellery completely, which was difficult for Elaine who had been a lover of silver jewellery since her teens and never took it off.

The ovaries and pituitary gland

Similar disturbances in the acupuncture points of the ovaries and pituitary gland would suggest possible problems relating to the menstrual cycle. Elaine did confirm this – her periods were rather erratic and she had started to suffer from night sweats. Assuming the menopause to be the cause of these irritating symptoms, she never gave them a second thought and just put up with them. Most people are unaware of the highly efficient lymphatic system within their body, which, if it breaks down, can lead to untold health problems. Congestion of this very important filtering system can quickly trigger or block sensors that carry messages all over the body. If the endocrine system happens to be the recipient of these out-of-tune signals, the range of unrelated symptoms could vary quite significantly. To reduce the risk of a hormonal imbalance it was necessary that Elaine's treatment should focus quite considerably on the pituitary gland and ovaries. It is worth mentioning here that ovarian cysts, and possibly appendicitis too, should be considered when a patient presents with a combination of disturbances similar to Elaine. The interactions of nerves associated with disturbance from the cervical ganglia and lymphatic congestion in the region of the intestines can cause chaos. First, there is usually an overtaxed drainage center, noticeably the lymphatic ducts, through tissue congestion and venous stasis. This is caused as a direct result of the congested cervical lymph nodes. Second, calcium production and absorption will be deficient if stimulus to the thyroid and parathyroid glands is incomplete. Third, calcium deposits will form quickly wherever there is reduced circulation of blood. The congested pelvic lymphatics often reflect the clogged thoracic duct and cistern with equal consequences: lymphatic and venous stasis, resulting in calcium deposits. Because of their association with the large number of lymph nodes in the vicinity, the appendix and the ovaries are often victims of the chaos, and medical intervention might be necessary.

The sympathetic nervous system

This system consists of a series of ganglia connected together by intervening cords, extending from the base of the skull to the coccyx. The system responds to 'fight or flight' situations; it produces increased heart and respiratory rates, increased blood flow to skeletal muscles, sweating and any other reaction that is associated with emergencies. The communications, which take place between two or more nerves, form a plexus. The abdominal area has many of these nerve plexuses, whose job it is to send nerve impulses all over the body.

The main abdominal plexus (the solar or epigastric plexus) supplies all the internal organs of the abdomen with a great network of nerves and ganglia, from its position behind the stomach but in front of the aorta (Pickford Pick & Howden 1988).

Abdominal massage works wonders here, draining the iliac and intestinal nodes, and reducing the risk of diverted nerve impulses away from the ovaries.

These nodes, which are often barely acknowledged by the therapist, have a tremendous task to perform, of cleansing and nourishing such a network of organs in the abdominal/pelvic region. Exercise 1 (lymph cistern) has many virtues, not least its direct influence upon the solar plexus and the intestines – in particular the duodenum and jejunum. Due to the congestion that Elaine experienced in these areas, peristalsis of the intestines would not have been sufficient to prevent sluggishness of the bowel. Sluggishness usually results in distension and another malfunction. Ultimately, a spasm forms in the intestines causing another area in the body with restricted access for nervous stimuli.

The duodenum is the first part of the small intestine, extending from the lower end of the stomach to the boundary of the jejunum. Ducts from the pancreas, liver, and gallbladder feed into the duodenum. The jejunum is the middle, coiled section of the small intestine. Whenever a spasm forms in either of these areas of the intestines it has become evident that spasm in abdominal muscles will shortly follow. When this happens, communications between the abdominal muscles and the nerve supply to the muscles of the upper spine and neck break down, causing muscle weakness and pain in the cervical region of the neck. If this condition is allowed to persist, the muscles of the upper spine and neck do not have the quality of nervous energy that is needed for health and stimulation. These muscles, which support the spine and head, cannot sustain the effort that is needed. This invariably causes strain, which eventually produces a spasm in the trapezius muscle and could ultimately develop into a frozen shoulder (see Chapter 10). In some instances, misalignment of the joints at the top of the spine occurs, with calcium deposits forming as a consequence. This is usually when the patient seeks help from the doctor. The majority of people with symptoms similar to these are suffering from congested lymphatic interactions with nerve plexus or ganglia within the body. The cause needs to be established and then the physiological faults can be corrected.

Symptoms of pain and discomfort in the upper spine and neck region can indeed respond to massage or manipulation. This can help the problem today, but it will be only a temporary help if the nerve supply is not corrected first. This can be put right by abdominal massage and Exercise 4 (the four-step exercise).

Abdominal massage frees the intestines of the spasm – not only does this allow the intestines to function normally, it also moves stagnant lymph and corrects the tone of the abdominal muscles, which permits all the nerves and signals from the epigastric plexus to flow freely. The muscles that support the head and neck will then receive the stimulus they need to do their job effectively. This massage alone can free many people from the pain and discomfort in the neck and upper spine region. Neck and shoulder massage followed by back massage will restore tone to the muscles and reduce the likelihood of calcium build-up. Reflexology to the filters and drainage points must follow any massage. The above explanation should dispel any confusion regarding abdominal massage when a patient complains of neck pain.

Metals that have been absorbed by the body can reach the intestinal tract with the bile, and can stick to the wall of the intestine adjacent to the ovary. This interference can distort nerve signals to the ovary and can quickly cause a malfunction (Martin 1990). It is always wise to check the lymphatics of the intestines and the inguinal lymph nodes if ovarian disruption is suspected. By maintaining a healthy intestinal tract, however, the patient will experience the real meaning of good health and avoid the many degenerative diseases that can be created here. Congestion of the abdominal lymphatics is often the core of disease due to the pathway of nerves that interweave this area, activating and stimulating the body. For this reason, abdominal massage is a prominent feature in this type of lymphatic drainage and in particular is an excellent way to assist in the correction of nerve impulses to the ovaries.

TREATMENT

Full details of how to perform the exercises in the following list can be found in Appendix 1.

1. **Reflexology.** To the liver, kidneys, spleen, lungs and lymph drainage points, followed by pituitary and thyroid glands and also the ovaries, and massage above and below the clavicles (see Fig. 9.1, pp 76–77).
2. **Exercise 1, lymph cistern.**
3. **Abdominal massage.**
4. **Exercise 4, the four-step exercise.**
5. **Exercise 2, lungs and upper abdomen.**
6. **Repeat Exercise 1, lymph cistern.**
7. **Do-in exercise.** Tap up along the center of the rib cage between the breasts, over each side, and then back down along the center.
8. **The rowing boat exercise.** This can be a bit difficult at first but is beneficial in helping to improve the nerve supply and tone to the muscles of the neck and upper spine.
9. **Red light massage.**
10. **Do-in.** Begin gentle tapping over the heart and sternum area.
11. **Reflexology.** To the liver, kidneys, spleen, lungs and lymph drainage points, large and

small intestines, thyroid and pituitary glands and ovaries. Finish this session: with the lymph cistern, liver, kidneys, spleen and lungs (see Fig. 9.1, pp 76–77).

It would be advisable to repeat this program every other day for 3 weeks. Thereafter once or twice a week as a lymphatic maintenance regime. Elaine assured me that she would start wearing rubber gloves whenever she was using any chemical substance in the future.

SECOND VISIT

Two weeks later Elaine returned, revealing the effects of the treatment. Upon leaving the clinic she said she had felt extremely cold. Two days later, just putting one foot in front of the other was difficult because her body ached all over. She suffered mood swings and her mouth was full of ulcers. Within 6 days of the treatment she started to feel better and, by 10 days, her neck problem became easier. She also identified an additional source of chlorine, that of neat bleach that she used to remove stains from tea and coffee cups at home and in the salon. Most cups and mugs are porous, therefore the next time the cup was used the drink would be nicely laced with chlorine.

Retesting of Elaine's acupuncture points showed an improvement in many areas of her body. She was not wearing any jewellery and wore gloves whenever she used perming and coloring solutions in the salon. Elaine's body had obviously decided to eliminate some of the toxic substances via her mouth and this was the reason for the mouth ulcers. The mood swings could also have occurred for the same reason but hormonal fluctuations should also be a consideration. Another factor is mental stress. Often, stress is brought about through worry or anxiety about one's family and Elaine's family problems hadn't disappeared. An overburdened lymphatic system will produce symptoms that many will be familiar with, such as sore throat or enlarged lymph nodes in the neck. Mood swings, however, don't usually fit into this category. It must be accepted that the human body cannot be broken into fragmented areas for treatment, rather it should be acknowledged as a complete unit where mind, body and spirit are not separated due to the relationship of lymph to almost every organ and tissue in the body. Lymph, together with the interconnection of energy fields, does not permit segregation, neither should any therapist.

There are disciplines that promote a positive mental approach and attitude in a patient, essentially to release tensions and stress. This is often difficult to sustain when the body is heavily congested with toxic matter that is distorting nerve impulses in all directions. Elaine was therefore advised to concentrate on cleansing her body for the time being. To continue with this program of cleansing would in the future be more advantageous to her family in view of the fact that it would allow her to eventually have a more positive outlook.

Chlorine was still evident in some of Elaine's acupuncture points and the source was found to be soap powder. She was using large amounts and the rinse cycle wasn't able to remove the excess powder. The amount of chlorine that can be absorbed from clothes, including bedclothes, can be quite significant. An eggcup full of soap powder is all that is required for an eight-pound load. Elaine also used bleach to clean her toilet and every day to clean the kitchen sink, all without gloves, as well as leaving the dishcloth soaking in bleach overnight. The high concentration of chlorine in liquid bleach was penetrating her body through her hands when she rinsed the cloth. Elaine was advised to wear rubber gloves at all times when handling bleach and to put her washing through a few extra rinse cycles, adding one tablespoon of bicarbonate of soda to her final rinse (bicarbonate of soda is the antidote to chlorine). This was done for at least 2 weeks to neutralize the chlorine in her clothes (Reed Gibson 2000).

Chlorine is a hormonal disrupter. Perhaps most patients would do well to avoid this chemical.

THIRD VISIT

Elaine returned some weeks later. Not only was she feeling considerably better, she was thrilled with the fact that she was saving substantial amounts of money on soap powder and bleach! On checking her points they revealed a much clearer body. The pain in her upper spine and neck was certainly much improved and she felt that she had a more positive outlook. Having once accepted night sweats as being part of the menopause, she was now less prepared to put up with the inconvenience.

Testing for food sensitivity revealed that milk, tea, coffee, sugar and orange juice should be avoided.

Each visit, abdominal massage was given as part of the treatment and every time it became less painful. On this third visit, however, it was evident that although Elaine's body was clearing well, she was still living under a lot of stress. Bach Flower Remedies were tested on this occasion, because of the length of time between appointments.

Bach Flower Remedies

Edward Bach began his career as a medical student at Birmingham University and then went on to the University College Hospital in London to complete his training. He qualified in 1912, gaining the Conjoint Diploma of MRCP, LRCP and, during the following year, gained the degrees of MB, BS and the Diploma of Public Health at Cambridge University.

During the course of his work, Bach became far more interested in the patients themselves than in their diseases. He would study the way they behaved, their outlook on life, their moods and emotions and he noted that those with an incentive to get well and with a cheerful outlook made far better progress than those who lacked that incentive or who were unhappy or hopeless. He began to see disease as an end product, a final stage, a physical manifestation of unhappiness, fear or worry (Howard 1987). He looked to nature for the answer and discovered 38 non-poisonous wild flowers.

Each of the 38 remedies is correlated to a specific negative state of mind, personality trait, mood or temperament that can often prove to be the real cause, psychosomatically, in the break down of one's physical and mental equilibrium (Ramsell 1986).

Elaine was tested with the remedies using ISR. Hornbeam and Pine gave positive tests. For this test the ATP spasm is not cleared prior to testing: instead it, and the magnetic field that it has created, are made use of. You will remember that the spasm will always form in the ATP muscle of a patient whenever the magnetic field of any substance is out of harmony with that person's own magnetic field. This also applies to hormones that the body produces during any emotional disturbance, and one can quickly assess the emotional stability of a patient using this method. When the Bach Flower Remedies are introduced into the patient's magnetic field, the remedy that reduces the muscle to its flaccid state is the one that is required. In this way, one can very quickly identify if an emotional disturbance is contributing to the patient's distorted magnetic fields. Harold Saxton Burr outlines many experiments on electrodynamic fields, or life fields, in *Blueprint for immortality*. In particular, he describes how abnormal voltage patterns can give warning of something out of shape in the body, well in advance of any actual symptoms:

Modern psychosomatic medicine has now demonstrated that, unfortunately, the effects of emotional disturbance are often not confined to mental symptoms: many physical ills have a psychosomatic origin. (Burr 1972, p 88)

Burr draws attention to the work of Dr Leonard J Ravitz Jr, at one time on the staff of the Department of Psychiatry at Yale. Ravitz's experiments and discovery 'that the state of the mind can affect the state of the field should induce a new sympathy for the emotionally distressed. Both emotional activity and stimuli of any sort involve mobilisation of electric energy. Hence, both emotions and stimuli evoke the same energy' (Burr 1972, p 89).

Often, more than one remedy will reduce the ATP muscle to its flaccid state when testing. These should be checked again with the patient holding all of the positive remedies at the same time. Elaine responded to hornbeam and pine. Dr Bach's interpretation of these remedies are as follows (Bach 1933):

- **Hornbeam:** *For those who feel that they have not sufficient strength, mentally or physically, to carry the burden of life placed upon them; the affairs of every day seem too much for them to accomplish, though they generally succeed in fulfilling their task ... for those who believe that some part, of mind or body, needs to be strengthened before they can easily fulfil their work.*
- **Pine:** *For those who blame themselves. Even when successful they think they could have done better, and are never content with their efforts or the results. They are hard working and suffer much from the faults they attach to themselves.*

These interpretations were given to Elaine, who was asked if they were correct. She was taken aback and agreed that they were, and was astonished at their accuracy of expression to what she was actually feeling. The two Bach Flower Remedies were included in her daily routine. Four drops were added to a drink four times a day. Elaine was also tested by way of ISR for vitamin and mineral supplements, plus nettle and sage teas.

Although Elaine still had personal problems, 4 weeks later her life had taken on a new meaning. The pain she was experiencing at the top of her spine and neck had almost disappeared. After 3 weeks of taking the Bach Flower Remedies she suddenly realized she hadn't taken any for a few days. This is just fine, as her body mustn't have needed them any more. The night sweats were not as bad either. She found that she continued to wake up but was able to go back to sleep quite quickly. Her tolerance levels also improved, which she accredited to the absence of pain.

FOURTH VISIT

Six months later, a more confident Elaine walked into the treatment room. She was convinced the night sweats were due to stress. They returned if she was upset, although they were not as bad as before the treatment. Elaine found that through understanding the reason behind the sweats, she was able to come through them quickly, especially with the help of the Bach Flower Remedies, which she left beside the bed to use when needed. Her faith in the remedies has led her to use her knowledge of them to help her son, until such time that he is able to accept professional help. Her overall improvement, hormonal included, meant that her tolerance level improved and she was able to look at things calmly, defusing situations before they developed into something extreme. Her ability to concentrate, understand and take in so much more has added to her self-confidence. As a result, Elaine gave up hairdressing and enrolled on a computing course. Luckily, the malfunctions in her body were corrected before any lasting damage had occurred. The practice of chemical and metal hygiene should be established by all, as prevention is better than cure.

Supplements

The supplements that Elaine found helpful are guaranteed 100% additive free (see Appendix 3 for suppliers). Tissue salts can be purchased from a health food store. Patients should, however, be encouraged to consult their GP before embarking on any supplementation.

- Vitamin E: 400 iu daily.
- B Forte Potency Vitamin B Complex: one a day.
- BioCaps: one a day.
- Evening Primrose Oil: 1000 mg daily.
- Nettle tea: two cups daily. This should not be prescribed for patients with high blood pressure.
- Miso: taken twice daily.
- Green tea: at least two cups daily.
- New Era Tissue Salts: Kali Phos for low energy.
- New Era Tissue Salts: Combination B for nervous exhaustion and general debility.
- Magnesium phosphate and calcium fluoride as tissue salts if there is inflammation.

Other household tips[1]

- **Bicarbonate of soda:** cleans teeth, works as a dry shampoo for pets and soothes mosquito

bites. An open box in the fridge dispels food smells for about 6 weeks and a handful added to a bath of lukewarm water will relieve the itching and pain of sunburn. A dirty pan filled with water and a teaspoon of bicarbonate of soda will cause food residues to lift off after half an hour. On a damp cloth it will clean glass oven doors – rub it over, leave to dry and polish with a soft cloth. Half a cupful scattered over the bottom of the dishwasher keeps it clean-smelling. It will also shine silver: make a paste, apply with a damp sponge, rinse off and polish.

- **Cream of tartar:** sprinkle some into washing water for whites, make a paste with water to remove brown smokestains. Used on a damp cloth it will clean and shine porcelain, and two teaspoons in a liter of water boiled in a stained saucepan will shine it up.

- **Glycerine:** wipe over bathroom mirrors to keep them fog free and add a tablespoon to the rinsing water to make woollens fluffy. It will keep washing pliable in the rinse and, when wiped over the freezer compartment, the next time it needs defrosting the ice will slip off in sheets.

- **Salt:** shake over oven spills as soon as they happen and when the oven cools the spill will brush off. Gargling with salt water is still probably the most popular old-fashioned remedy for a sore throat.

- **Sugar:** can help keep flowers fresh; add a little to the water in a vase. Keep biscuits crisp by putting a cube in the tin.

- **Tea:** can be employed as a stain for furniture; brush a strong brew over old pine furniture to give it an antique look.

- **Vinegar:** will absorb smells; a bowl left in a freshly painted room will dispel the odor in a day. A few drops of vinegar can be added to the washing up water. Wiped over the inside of a fridge it discourages mildew and a weak solution can be used for cleaning glass and windows.

- **Hydrogen peroxide:** is to be found in the cells of the body. It is created there from water and oxygen and acts as a major defense in the immune system. It is produced in healthy individuals in sufficient quantity to counteract unwanted bacterial invaders (Pitchford 1993, p 40).

---

[1] Taken from recommendations published by the Allergy and Chemical Sensitivity Association of South Australia

In the kitchen, hydrogen peroxide (H_2O_2 3% = volume 10) can be used as an antiseptic. Other uses are:
- vegetable soak: add $\frac{1}{4}$ cup H_2O_2 to a sink full of cold water. Soak light vegetables (lettuce, etc.) for 20 minutes; thicker-skinned vegetables (like cucumbers) for 30 minutes. Drain and dry (they will also keep longer)
- leftover tossed salad: put 1 tablespoon H_2O_2 in $\frac{1}{2}$ cup of water and spray the top of the salad with the solution before covering and refrigerating. An added tip is to put the salad (including tomatoes, radishes, etc.) in the blender with $\frac{1}{2}$ cup of juiced tomato,

carrot, etc. Blend, then fold in additional $\frac{1}{2}$ cup of juice. Add seasoning to taste
- washing: add 8 oz H_2O_2 to your washing in place of bleach
- plants: put 1 oz H_2O_2 in 2 pints of water. Water or mist with this solution to aid growth
- as an insecticide spray: add 8 oz of white sugar and 4–8 oz of 3% H_2O_2 to 1 gallon of water.

The reflexology charts and acupuncture points that are relevant for this case study are shown in Figs 9.1 and 9.2 and are to be used in conjunction with ISR and lymphatic drainage techniques.

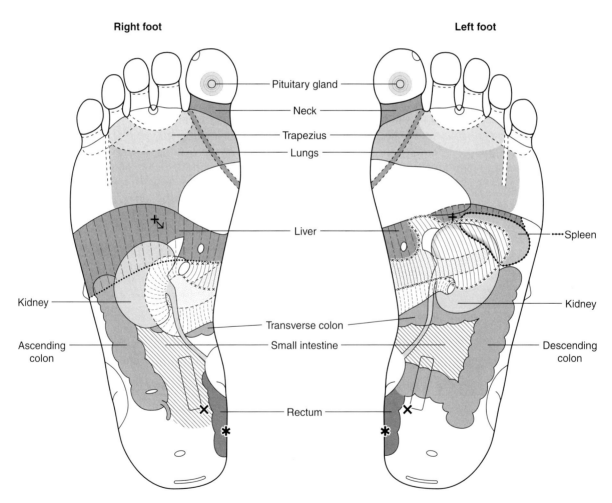

Figure 9.1 Reflexology chart for the liver, kidneys, spleen, lungs, lymph drainage points, large and small intestines, thyroid gland, pituitary gland and ovaries (the trapezius and neck can also be massaged if needed). © F. Fox, used with permission.

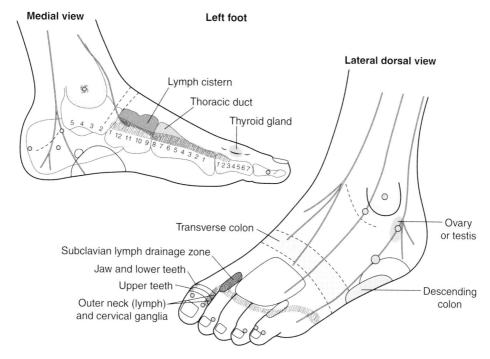

Figure 9.1 (*continued*). Unless otherwise stated, all reflex zones apply to both feet.

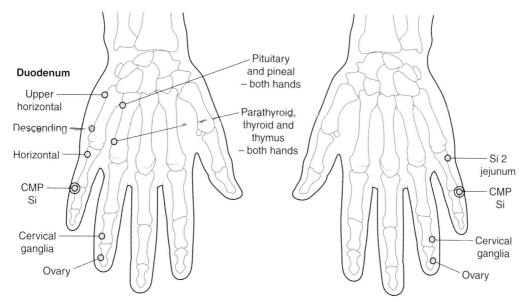

Figure 9.2 Relevant acupuncture points. The points illustrated are for fingertip testing, assessment, and acupressure only. CMP, control measurement point.

REFERENCES

Bach E 1933 The twelve healers and other remedies.
C W Daniels, Saffron Walden
Burr H S 1972 Blueprint for immortality – the electric
patterns of life. C W Daniels, Saffron Walden
Howard J 1987 The story of Mount Vernon. The Edward
Bach Foundation, Oxfordshire, UK, p 7
Martin S 1990 Mercury is it your problem? Here's health;
September
Pickering Pick T, Howden R 1988 Gray's Anatomy
(Classic Collector's edition). Crown Publishers,
UK, p 1082
Pitchford P 1993 Healing with whole food. North Atlantic
Books, Berkeley, California, p 40
Ramsell J 1991 Questions & answers: the Bach flower
remedies. C W Daniels, Saffron Walden, p 11
Reed Gibson P Multiple chemical sensitivity.
New Harbinger Publications Inc, America, pp 53–54

FURTHER READING

Howard J, Ramsell J 1990 The original Writings of Edward
Bach. C W Daniels, Saffron Walden
McKenzie R 1983 Treat your own neck. Spinal Publications
Ltd, New Zealand
Ramsell J 1986 Questions and answers: the Bach flower
remedies. C W Daniels, Saffron Walden
Weeks N 1940 The medical studies of Edward Bach.
C W Daniels, Saffron Walden

10

Frozen shoulder

This is a continuation of Stephen's case study, which was described in Chapter 6. It has been included to illustrate the intricacy of the interconnecting energy fields. This case study shows perfectly the research behind this particular integrated therapy and illustrates how distorting energy from one ganglia or plexus will affect another seemingly unconnected part of the body. When a patient presents with a frozen shoulder an attentive therapist should bear in mind that the problem could arise from a stomach problem or allergic reaction, and should check the energy field of the celiac plexus. Chapter 6 showed that formaldehyde and medication had contributed to Stephen's lower back problems, which responded to lymphatic drainage techniques. In addition, he was tested for food sensitivity, with the result that tea, milk, wheat and coffee should be avoided.

On numerous occasions when a frozen shoulder has been diagnosed, particularly the right shoulder, the celiac plexus will register a low energy reading, as will the ascending colon and duodenum. The celiac plexus is a direct continuation from the solar plexus and subdivides into the gastric, hepatic and splenic plexuses. The gastric plexus, which is located on the artery that supplies the stomach, provides the main autonomic nerve supply to the stomach.

FOURTH VISIT

Stephen's acupuncture points were tested in more detail to find the precise areas of

congestion. The pit of the stomach registered a very low energy – this is usually where ulcers form – the pylorus was also low in energy. Formaldehyde and substances contained within the medication Stephen was taking were also identified in these areas. The pylorus is the lower outlet from the stomach to the duodenum. When a narrowing of this outlet occurs it obstructs the passage of food into the duodenum. In adults such narrowing can be the result of scarring from peptic ulcers. When this condition is medically diagnosed, surgery is normally required whereby the outlet is widened to ensure the free passage of food into the intestine. However, investigations would appear to suggest that the narrowing of this outlet in adults is the result of lymphatic congestion. The stomach has numerous lymph vessels in and on its wall and a substantial number of nodes, particularly around the cardiac and pyloric ends. Lymph drained from the stomach will eventually be collected by the celiac nodes, which lie in front of the aorta. The stomach, therefore, is dependent upon these lymph vessels functioning correctly. However, when the body is faced with a substance that it cannot tolerate, including food, it will respond to the invasion by trying to get rid of it as quickly as possible. This often produces gas in the stomach, and its ability to expand in this way means that continuous compression can be placed upon the tissues and the many blood and lymph vessels associated in and around the stomach, restricting lymph and venous flow. Medication, in particular salicylic acid (from aspirin), does appear to stick to the wall of the pylorus and either obstructs the exit or limits the vibrational energy. When the stomach is empty the pylorus is situated just to the right of the median line of the body, on a level with the upper border of the first lumbar vertebra. As the stomach becomes distended the pylorus moves to the right and, in a fully distended stomach, can be situated two or three inches to the right of the median line. The two most important acupuncture points to check for problems associated with the stomach are the pit of the stomach and pylorus: St 43 on the lateral side of the proximal epicondyle of the second metatarsal of the right foot and St 45 the terminal point on the lateral side of the second toe of the right foot.

The final part of the treatment on this fourth visit consisted of a stomach wash, which must only be performed on an empty stomach. This must not be carried out if the patient is experiencing reflux, the presence of any blood in the stool, severe pain or under medical supervision without their doctor's consent.

Stomach wash

As this procedure needs to be carried out on an empty stomach, the patient will need prior notice not to eat anything for 3 hours before commencement of the treatment.

The patient should be given a large glass of filtered water to drink. They should then lie on the treatment couch where reflexology to the filters and lymph drainage points must be given for about 5 minutes, followed by massage above and below the clavicles.

Begin the procedure with gentle massage of the abdomen in relation to the celiac axis, then palpate into the splenic flexure where the splenic nodes receive a part of the stomach's lymph along the splenic artery. This might produce some discomfort for the patient. Providing the discomfort is moderate and not a sharp pain, proceed to palpate this area until the gurgling of the water in the stomach can be heard. Continue with this manipulation for a short time, observing the patient for any discomfort. Sustaining this gentle procedure will encourage any substance

that is sticking to the wall of the stomach to detach itself, removing the focus. Often, a gurgle can be heard, which heralds the water's exit from the stomach via the pylorus into the duodenum, taking with it any substance that was distorting the energy. The patient must then roll onto his or her right side for 3 minutes, to allow the rest of the water to drain into the duodenum. Once there, the webbing between the thumb and finger of the right hand can be checked for a spasm, giving the opportunity for the antagonistic material from the stomach/pylorus to be identified. Wait 3 minutes before returning the patient to the supine position and palpate into the hepatic flexure for a few moments, before asking the patient to turn onto the left side for a further 3 minutes. Return once more to the supine position and further palpate the duodenum area, this time to encourage the water and contents to flow freely through the intestines. Normal abdominal massage should now be undertaken, with the emphasis on the small intestine. It is quite fascinating for the therapist when this procedure is completed to observe the patient check the improved mobility of the previously frozen joint and instant relief. The therapist should verify the impact of this massage on the acupuncture points for the celiac plexus, stomach, colon and small intestine to appreciate the power of this physical therapy. The procedure should finish with reflexology to the liver, kidneys, spleen, lung, lymph drainage points, stomach and pylorus.

This absence of pain, however, could be short lived, as it will depend upon the amount of toxic matter remaining within the lymph nodes, the lining of the stomach and pylorus. For this reason, patient participation is strongly encouraged and it is the responsibility of the therapist to guide and support the patient on the intricacies of the technique so that it can be performed each morning before getting out of bed. This procedure is ongoing until the congested areas are clear of toxins and the flow of energy has been re-established. Together with the exclusion of food sensitivities from the diet, the patient will experience a gradual reduction of pain. An established routine that accommodates these integrated therapy techniques will need to be practised for a period of time.

FIFTH VISIT

A month later Stephen's back had greatly improved and he had started to work in the garden again, although he did have to be careful not to bend over for long periods or lift anything heavy. He discovered that arduous car journeys were achievable once more, provided his exercises could be accomplished en route, otherwise he would be very stiff on reaching his destination. He was advised to replace his manual car with an automatic one as soon as possible. This is actually very good advice for any back pain suffer, as the muscles of the legs, spine and also the psoas muscles become taut whilst maintaining the driving position required in a car with a manual gear box. Consequently, any existing spinal condition will inevitably be at risk as often the weight of the body will be borne by the sides of the buttocks while driving instead of by the ischial tuberosities. Stephen had actually dispensed with all of his medication and was thrilled that his stomach problem had improved immensely within 8 days of following his restricted diet.

The frozen shoulder had returned within 4 days of his previous treatment. By his own admission, Stephen became complacent after the last treatment when the pain disappeared and didn't continue with the stomach wash. However, once he included it in his morning routine, he found that the pain disappeared again. The presence of the pain prompted him back to the necessity of the routine. This treatment session continued much the same as the previous two.

SIXTH VISIT

After 2 months, Stephen was much improved. He was delighted with the results he'd achieved through the treatment program and grateful that he had been given the chance to help himself. Most of his exercises had become a part of his routine but needed to be performed only twice a

week to keep everything under control and pain free. He has become meticulous in his dealings with chemicals and takes every precaution to avoid inhalation and absorbency. The following exercise program formed Stephen's treatment sessions on his last two visits. The therapist will be familiar with all of the moves and might like to pass the patient guide on to assist with patient participation of the therapy.

Patient guide

Appendix 2 contains instructions to the patient on how to perform the exercises in the following list.

1. **Reflexology:**
(i) liver, kidneys, spleen, lungs and lymph drainage points (see Fig. 10.2, pp 84–85).
(ii) massage above and below the clavicles.
I would recommend that these two procedures be carried out for 3 weeks prior to the exercise program and stomach wash.
2. **Stomach wash.** When the stomach is empty (preferably before getting out of bed in the morning), drink a glass of water, wait a few minutes then lie on your back. With the tips of your fingers gently, palpate under the sternum and to the left of the rib cage (Fig. 10.1a), until you hear the water gurgling. Then lie on your right side for 3 minutes, before returning to your back, where you palpate under the right side of the rib cage (Fig. 10.1b). Again, you might hear the water. Turn on to your left side for 3 minutes, then onto your back once more, where you palpate under the left side of the ribs down to the waist area (Fig. 10.1c). This also helps to clear the mesenteric plexus, which could help with constipation.
3. **Reflexology.** To the liver, kidneys, spleen, lungs, lymph drainage points, stomach, pylorus (see Fig. 10.2, pp 84–85).
4. **Self-help abdominal massage.**
5. **Exercise 1, lymph cistern.**

It may be wise for the patient to continue with the above program for 4 weeks before embarking on any further exercises. You must remember to conclude any program with reflexology to the

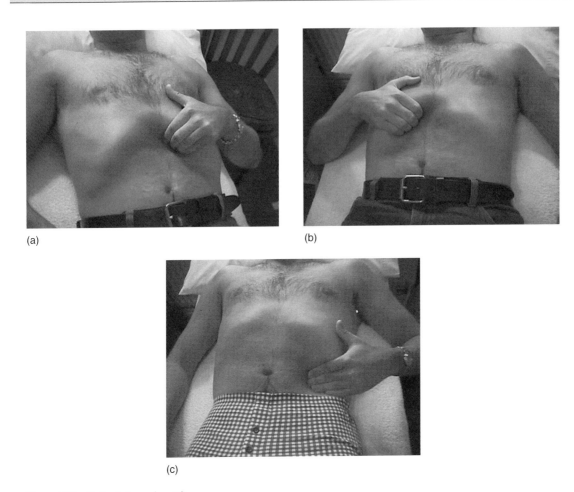

(a)

(b)

(c)

Figure 10.1 Patient stomach wash.

liver, kidneys, spleen, lungs and lymph drainage points.

6. **Exercise 4, the four-step exercise.** This helps to stimulate the nerve supplies of the celiac plexus, abdominal aortic plexus, solar plexus, duodenum and jejunum, and decongests the superior mesenteric lymph nodes in the epigastrium. This is best performed by the patient under the guidance of the therapist but can be repeated at home.

7. **The red light exercise.**
8. **The rowing boat exercise.**
9. **Repeat Exercise 1, lymph cistern.**
10. **Do-in.** Gently over the whole of the chest and thyroid area.
11. **Reflexology.** To the liver, kidneys, spleen, lungs, lymph drainage points, pancreas, stomach, pylorus, small and large intestines and lymph cistern (see Fig. 10.2, pp 84–85).

Stephen recovered quite quickly from his frozen shoulder, due in part to the previous treatments that he received for his back problem. For this reason, do not loose heart if your frozen shoulder takes a little longer to respond. Follow the treatment program and, provided that no other area of the body is congested, you too should recover in time. It is recommended that reflexology be carried out for 3 weeks prior to the exercises and stomach wash. Stephen was advised to avoid all caffeine (he was sensitive to coffee) as it would further aggravate his stomach problems: caffeine is an alkaloid found in coffee, chocolate, tea and cola.

It is a central nervous system stimulant, which increases the rate of metabolism and triggers the release of stress hormones. These increase the heart rate and blood pressure, and the use of oxygen and vitamins. Hypermetabolism uses up vitamins more quickly, especially vitamins B1, B2 and niacin, which is needed to supply extra glucose. In responding to stress, the adrenal glands also require extra vitamin C, B5 and choline. In excess, caffeine depletes the body of B complex vitamins, especially B1, B5 and B6. This could lead to anxiety, hyperactivity, insomnia, irritability, and cardiovascular weakness. Loss of niacin and B2 can lead to stomach and muscle weakness. At the same time, caffeine can act as a diuretic, leading to loss of important minerals (Fox, unpublished work).

Stephen responded to the following homeopathic remedies and tissue salts, all of which can be purchased in health stores:

- New Era tissue salts combination C: for acidity and heartburn.
- New Era magnesium phosphate: to soothe the system.
- Calcium carbonate: settles the stomach.
- Lachesis: helps support the pylorus, ileo-cecal valve and rectal muscles while healing takes place.
- Bicarbonate of soda B.P. $\frac{1}{4}$ teaspoon in a glass of cooled boiled water will reduce the stomach acid (no more than twice a day). If symptoms persist for more than a week then see your doctor.

- Honey: 1 teaspoon in a glass of hot water before going to bed can be very soothing.
- Medicinal charcoal tablets and biscuits: can settle an over-acid stomach and relieve nausea (especially during cancer treatment).
- Miso: each morning, on an empty stomach.

Back pain accompanied by frozen shoulder is a common occurrence. It is therefore possible to combine the exercises outlined in this chapter and in Chapter 6 if you suffer similar symptoms. However, it is not advisable to do the combined exercises all at once. Your therapist will be able to advise you but I would recommend any patient to follow the reflexology chart for 3 weeks, then proceed with the back pain treatment before introducing the remaining exercises to treat a frozen shoulder.

EXERCISE

It is a fallacy that a bad back needs rest – it needs exercise. It is also a fallacy to suggest that swimming can be beneficial for back pain. Many back pain sufferers dutifully swim and make themselves worse. Listen to your body and, if it hurts, stop. If you do swim, remember to allow at least 5 minutes in the shower afterwards to wash the chlorine from your hair and body.

The reflexology charts and acupuncture points that are relevant for this case study are shown in Figs 10.2 and 10.3 and are to be used in conjunction with ISR in association with the particular lymphatic drainage techniques for integrated therapy.

Right foot

Left foot

Neck

Lungs

Shoulder

Shoulder

Stomach
×××

Liver

Spleen

Pylorus

×××Stomach×××

Pancreas

Kidney

Kidney

Transverse colon

Ascending
colon

Small intestine

Descending
colon

Rectum

Figure 10.2 Reflexology chart for the liver, kidneys, spleen, lungs, lymph drainage points, pancreas, stomach, pylorus, intestines and lymph cistern. © F. Fox, used with permission.

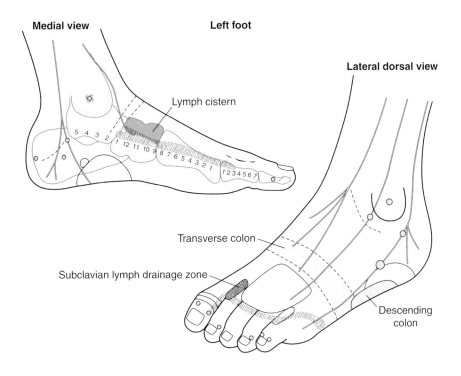

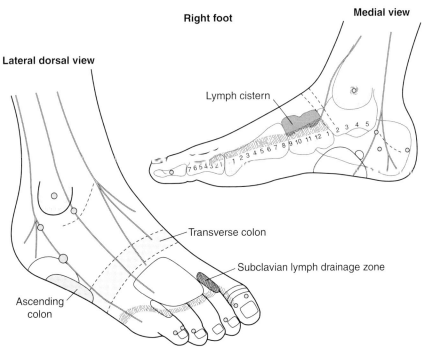

Figure 10.2 (*continued*).

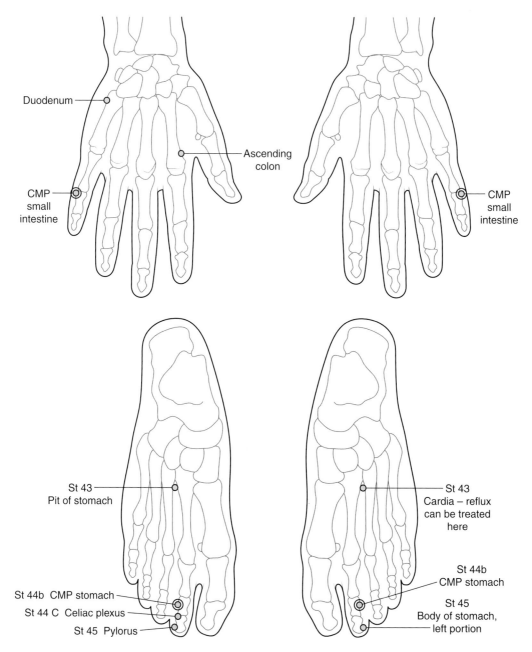

Figure 10.3 Relevant acupuncture points. The points illustrated are for fingertip testing, assessment, and acupressure only.

11

Mercury sensitivity

FIRST VISIT

Angela presented with a host of symptoms: aches and pains in her joints; legs that were varicose, often inflamed and felt like lead; and extremely bad headaches. She also found it difficult to focus on objects and generally felt under the weather.

Angela was a housewife living abroad, with a husband, three children and various animals to look after. Her life was very busy, especially as all members of the family had a 2-hour lunch break, which they took at home. Whether by tradition or design, Angela cooked both at lunchtime and in the evening for all the family. The family home was very close to the center of town where Angela did most of her shopping. Walking into town had once been enjoyable but was now becoming a problem. The pain she experienced in her shoulders made carrying the bags of food difficult and the routine was causing fatigue. She suffered from constant colds, which were not helped by the usual cold preparations. A visit to the doctor for a blood test revealed no abnormalities and the prescribed antibiotics did not have any effect.

Testing Angela's acupuncture points revealed a combination of metals – silver, mercury, zinc and nickel, but mostly mercury.

This combination of metals is usually consistent with silver amalgam fillings in the teeth. Fillings are composed of 50% metallic mercury, 35% silver, 9% tin, 6% copper, and a trace of zinc.[1]

Angela had recently been to the dentist for a check up and to have her teeth cleaned. Everything had been satisfactory.

Taking previous experience into account, and given the low energy reading from the acupuncture points, there was a considerable amount of amalgam in the body. This presented a problem as mercury in particular is not an easy substance to eliminate and Angela was not able to come to regular treatment sessions.

Under normal circumstances, a return visit to the dentist would be recommended to determine if one of the fillings was leaking, and to remove the faulty filling if this was the case. Under no circumstances should there be any cutting of corners in the extensive preparations for this procedure. As the amount of amalgam that is released when the dentist drills a filling is quite significant, and as the debris will fly in all directions, every attempt should be made not only to protect the mucous membrane of the nose and throat, but also the rest of the body. The response of the nose and throat to any irritation would be to secrete mucus in an attempt to wash away the irritant. This can be easily identified and rectified by blowing the nose.

---

[1] As explained in the introductory section, entitled 'Dental amalgam issue', of the website: www.amalgam.org

Unfortunately, once the irritant substance hits the lymph nodes in the neck, they will quickly become congested if the vessels and nodes are unable to accommodate the attempt to neutralize the irritant. The resulting congestion will inevitably set off a chain reaction that becomes very apparent as a consequence of stifled interconnecting energy fields, and which cannot be rectified by simply blowing the nose. As the lymphatic vessels become compounded by this steady flow of metal-laden mucus, the excess spills into the tissues (because it has nowhere else to drain to) and will wind its way deeper into the body. To prevent this penetration it is vitally important that, at the point of entry, lymphatic vessels can accommodate the increased load and deal effectively with the swift removal of the irritant from the body. In essence, a program of lymph drainage exercises, which serve to produce harmonious oscillations between organs and tissues, needs to be completed to a satisfactory level to achieve this goal. Not to do this could cause a catalog of health problems.

Unfortunately, Angela's schedule didn't allow sufficient time for this preparation. It is quite extensive and arduous, and includes careful screening of the filters while the existing metals are removed from the lymphatic system. The heart and lungs are vulnerable at this stage of lymphatic drainage and therefore must be checked and rechecked to prevent any old mercury attaching itself to the lymphatics of these organs. There is no given timescale for this preparation, it is solely dependent upon the depth of pollution within that body and its ability to remove the debris. An already disabled nervous system struggling with the removal of amalgam could take months to regain the correct stimuli to prevent inappropriate interactions of the energy fields and at the same time gain sufficient energy that is required to discard this rubbish. Although it is of paramount importance to remove the source of the mercury as quickly as possible, i.e. the filling, on this occasion it was not safe to do so.

There are dentists who are familiar with the dangers of amalgam removal and who take every precaution available to them, but the body will still absorb toxic fumes and particles while the filling

is being removed. The particles of metal that accumulate in the mouth as a result should be a matter of great concern. They do penetrate the body and the standard procedures that are in place to prevent such an occurrence are grossly inadequate.

Some dental and medical professionals believe that metals such as mercury are absorbed directly into the bloodstream when any corrosion takes place, and that from the bloodstream they are filtered out by the kidneys to escape with urine. Therefore, the standard clinical test for mercury and other metal poisoning is analysis of the blood or urine; blood tests are used to determine mercury sensitivity and whether mercury is leaking into the body. Indeed, the following appears on the internet site www.dentistzone.com:

Amalgam-related illness: frequently asked questions (FAQ). We know that:

- Dental amalgam fillings consist of 50% mercury
- Mercury leaks from the fillings
- Mercury is highly toxic and
- Low grade chronic mercury intoxication can give rise to symptoms such as anxiety, irritability, fatigue, outbursts of temper, stress intolerance, decreased simultaneous capacity, loss of self-confidence, indecision, headache, depression, metallic taste, etc.

Thus, amalgam-related illness is accepted by the medical profession, which remains unclear as to how to eliminate this dangerous substance from the body.

After completing years of trials Fox argued that 'analysis of the blood or urine is usually inadequate because many problems arise from metals in the lymphatics, before they enter the bloodstream' (Fox, unpublished work, 1988). According to his findings, the normal route of excretion is via the liver and bile system into the intestinal tract and thence from the body. Hence blood and urine tests for evidence of mercury or other metal poisoning are inadequate. Only when the liver becomes overloaded with such metals and can no longer filter them effectively from the blood do the kidneys become involved. It would appear that mercury and other metals build up in the tissues of the mouth and jaw and are then absorbed by the network of lymphatic capillaries in the mouth. There are many routes that mercury and other metals can take from this starting point in the mouth and they can build up quite a presence in the lymphatics of the lungs and heart, the mammary glands, intestinal tracts and many other organs. Eventually, even the inguinal lymph nodes can become clogged with metals that originate in the mouth, causing interference with the circulatory system in pelvic organs and the legs.

In 1987 Fox stumbled upon something quite remarkable while he was using a medical magnet; for this reason he called this magnet the 'super snooper'. The magnet was originally designed to be used in conjunction with the Mora therapy machine and was never considered for any additional use. However, Fox discovered quite by accident that the magnet could be used to identify toxic substances outside the body that were responsible for contributing to low acupuncture point readings (see Chapter 13). He also discovered that metals could be tracked and the routes mapped as they leaked into the body: not all metals take exactly the same route or adhere to the same areas of the body, but generally they enter the body through the skin and then the lymphatics of the gums and cheeks. They pass down through these lymphatics, through the deep lymphatics of the neck to the two lymph drainage points and into the subclavian vein. Once the deep lymphatics of the neck are congested with metals, the lymph drainage of the sinuses, eyes and ears will undoubtedly be impaired. The mucous membranes will increase their secretions in an attempt to address the situation, which intensifies the congestion. Problems such as sinusitis, impaired vision and hearing can develop in this area as a result. Sometimes mercury, and other metals, will enter nerve fibers in the gums and take a different route, working their way up through a cranial nerve to the brain. The serious ramifications of brain wave function described by Oschman (2000, p 96) must be considered in

regard to metals in the mouth: that is, that brain waves are not constant in frequency and vary from moment to moment (Oschman 2000). Research has indicated that the brain has a 'silent phase', which lasts from 5 to 25 seconds, and it is probably at this time that the brain is susceptible to external vibrations. The electroencephalographic waves spread not only throughout the brain but throughout the whole nervous system and into every part of the organism regulating the activity of the entire nervous system. Depressive conditions and illness emanating from the brain could therefore originate in the mouth. Mercury that is inhaled and swallowed can work its way up through the lymphatics of the lungs, stomach and esophagus towards the lymph drainage points, from where it can congest the lymphatics of the heart.

The divergence of conditions associated with malfunctioning energy fields and impaired circulation of tissue fluid in the heart muscle could lead to degeneration of heart tissue, eventually triggering a heart attack. As heart tissue breaks up, it causes a pool of blood, which backs up into the coronary artery and can give the appearance of coronary thrombosis. But the clot of blood in the coronary artery is the *result* of a heart attack, not its cause. Chronic congestion of the lymph drainage of the heart usually goes undetected and is practically undiagnosable apart from EAV and ISR. Hence the large number of unexpected heart attacks despite strict medical supervision. Discussions of this topic are prolific on the internet. Indeed, at www.amalgam.org, you will find an article entitled *Mercury associated with cardiac dysfunction* (Frustaci et al 1999), which discusses the possibility of a link between the two, although it is not understood *why* there is a link. Research undertaken over many years by Fox and myself using EAV discovered a link.

As the lymph drains into the subclavian veins it goes directly to the right side of the heart, then through the capillary beds of the lungs and returns to the left side of the heart before passing into general circulation. The heart and lungs are vulnerable if the lymph is full of mucous and toxic waste, in particular metals such as mercury. These metals serve as signals that deactivate the circuitry of the body's natural communications.

The possibility of a heart attack, therefore, must never be taken lightly in a patient with a heavily congested lymphatic system, particularly one laden with metals. Integrated therapy with its emphasis on physical therapy can correct any physiological faults and restore to normal the disturbed energy fields. This will allow the integrated processes of growth, repair and defense; in fact it caters for the complete function of the organism as a whole.

According to Voll, lymphatic stasis (blockage) in the heart is a substantial prerequisite for heart failure and infarct (localized area of dead tissue resulting from obstruction of the blood supply to that part) (Voll 1984). Sweden banned the use of mercury on pregnant women in 1990 because of fears that a developing fetus is vulnerable to its toxicity (*Daily Mail* 1990). Some years later, the British government also announced that pregnant women should not receive amalgam fillings, for fear that mercury could cross the placenta and damage the fetus. Before amalgam can cross the placenta to the fetus, it must first enter the mothers' bloodstream, thereby polluting her body first.

As early as 1926 there was doubt as to the use of amalgam fillings. Professor Dr Alfred Stock, from the Kaiser-Wilhelm Institute of Chemistry wrote (Ziff 1984, p 11):

Dentistry should completely avoid the use of amalgam for fillings, or at least not use it whenever this is possible. There is no doubt that many symptoms: tiredness, depression, irritability, vertigo, weak memory, mouth inflammations, diarrhoea, loss of appetite and chronic catarrhs, are often caused by mercury, which the body is exposed to from amalgam fillings in small amounts, but continuously. Doctors should give this fact their serious consideration. It will then likely be found that the thoughtless introduction of amalgam as a filling material for teeth was a severe sin against humanity.

Professor Stock went on to publish an article in 1939 outlining further facts about amalgam: he identified it as 'an unstable alloy that continuously gave off mercury in the form of gas ions and abraded particles' (Ziff 1984). These serious allegations were delivered many years ago and yet mercury continues to be used in the material for filling teeth.

The toxic time bomb (Ziff 1984) highlights still further the dangers of amalgam fillings:

There is no such thing as a stable amalgam filling. Each one will leak mercury in every direction; into the body of the tooth, into the gum tissue surrounding the tooth and bone, into the air of the mouth, where it is carried to the nose and brain, and into saliva where it is both carried as mercury into the bloodstream and methylated by normal body bacteria into the dangerous poison methylmercury. We are dealing with a known and proven poison ... Based upon the current documented scientific knowledge and research, a dentist cannot, with impunity, introduce a metal into a patient's mouth and expect there to be no biological effect ... Numerous documented studies show that the introduction of silver–mercury amalgam filling will cause leakage of mercury into the body. The later use of gold or palladium alloy elsewhere in the mouth will cause the more rapid release of mercury.

Degenerative diseases are increasing, year on year, despite the money that is spent on research and drugs. Yet the lymphatic system, which holds many clues, is still virtually untapped and ignored as a vast store of information into the causes of these debilitating disorders. ISR can identify the areas of congestion within the body, together with their source, and can be used not only in the prevention of these degenerative diseases but as a restorative for the immune system.

When lymph is examined under the microscope, white blood cells called lymphocytes are seen floating in the transparent fluid. These are always increased in number after the passage of the lymph through lymphoid tissue, as in the lymphatic glands. They are constantly furnishing a fresh supply of colorless corpuscles to the blood (Pickering Pick & Howden 1988, p 1082).

Lymphocytes migrate through the blood to lymphatic tissue, where they proliferate and produce more lymphocytes, which are the core of our immune system. They are responsible for destroying microorganisms and controlling tumors. Lymphocytes make up about 25% of the blood's white cells and give the body its natural immunity to disease. They do this by making antitoxins to counteract the potentially damaging effects of the powerful poisons or chemicals produced by some bacteria. The other essential tasks of the lymphocytes are to make antibodies and chemicals that help prevent body cells from succumbing to bacterial invasion.

Lymphocytes develop into two types of cells. The first type, which makes antibodies, is known as the B lymphocyte, or B cell. The second, identical in appearance but with a different function, is known as the T cell. T cells produced in the lymph nodes are alerted to attack foreign tissue and viruses by helper cells, which carry messages of invasion to developing lymphocytes. These develop a chemical memory of the specific protein, or antigen, of the invader, and, should it enter the body again, the lymphocytes can recognize and then destroy them. In this way the body builds up an immunity to specific viruses (Horton 1985).

The following text comes from a research report written by Dr David Eggleston (1984):

Removing 6 amalgam restorations increased the T-lymphocyte percentage from 47% (before removal) to 73% (after removal). Preliminary data suggest that dental amalgam and dental nickel alloys can adversely affect the quantity of T-lymphocytes.

Looking closely at this evidence it would appear that the percentage increase of T lymphocytes would have increased still further if lymphatic drainage had been introduced prior to the removal of amalgam fillings. This research would suggest that physical therapy of the type that promotes and encourages movement of lymph through tissue and nodes must surely become part of the body's defense and repair mechanism. By manipulating and balancing the vibratory circuits (Oschman 2000) in this way, the unobstructed flow of electrical energy through the tissues would generate the power that is essential for prevention and for just feeling well.

Treatment

It is crucial for the health of the patient that during the treatment sessions the therapist is aware of any congestion to the lymphatics of the heart and lungs. These areas should be monitored carefully.

1. **Reflexology.** To the liver, kidneys, spleen, heart, lungs and lymph drainage points (see Fig. 11.1, p 100).

2. **Massage.** Above and below the clavicles.

The patient must drink eight glasses of water a day.

Angela was given a chart for these areas with a recommendation that she repeat this procedure each night for one week. In addition, the mineral selenium was recommended, which is the antidote to mercury.[2] Angela responded favorably to this when her body was challenged using ISR and one tablet each day for a week was suggested.

Selenium is usually combined with vitamins A, C and E. It appears to attach itself to mercury in the body, which in turn allows for a swifter decongestion of those polluted areas. However, this must only be used for a short time, as an aid to elimination. Overuse in the presence of existing fillings could draw mercury from the fillings into the body.

SECOND VISIT

Angela attended 1 week later. She had suffered a severe headache just 12 hours after the treatment, followed by diarrhea on the next day. This reaction is quite common when the body is so highly polluted with toxic substances. It is the body's way of expressing its eagerness to expel the toxin as quickly as possible and demonstrates just how powerful reflexology can be and the importance of preparatory involvement prior to amalgam removal.

After 5 days of reflexology, the acupuncture points for the kidneys had greatly improved, but not all of the other organs had responded equally. On retesting the kidneys, the reading had changed and was lower! Angela was wearing her

---

[2] After extensive research, Fox discovered that the antidote for mercury in biophysics is selenium. In 1980, this was confirmed by Kristensen and Hansen (Ziff 1984, pp 44 and 146).

skirt when the kidneys were tested originally, but had removed her skirt prior to massage before the second reading. Angela was to visit a friend after her appointment and she had put her selenium tablet in her skirt pocket, intending to take it after her lunch. However, when the selenium was in close contact with the body as opposed to being ingested, the acupuncture point for the kidneys and many other areas of the body improved! This was tested by taping the capsule on to Angela's body between her shoulder blades in the region of T2 (because the sympathetic innervation is shared with the thymus).

Because of the danger in releasing too much mercury from tissues, it is important to take this treatment slowly – particularly because of the impact that mercury can have on the heart and lungs. Therefore, abdominal massage could be introduced in this second treatment along with the homeopathic remedy Viscum Alb.6c, which Angela responded to using ISR. The need for caution was still a priority, for this reason reflexology remained the focal point in Angela's treatment.

Treatment

1. **Reflexology.** To the liver, kidneys, spleen, heart, lungs, lymph drainage points and pancreas (see Fig. 10.2). Massage above and below both clavicles.

2. **Abdominal massage.**

3. **Relexology.** To the liver, kidneys, spleen, heart and lungs.

It would be advisable to have the patient repeat this treatment program each evening and to drink eight glasses of water each day.

THIRD VISIT

After 5 days Angela again was pleased to report that she had not suffered from any reaction to the previous treatment. She was still drinking eight glasses of water a day and continuing to follow her chart for reflexology. The selenium tablet, which she was still taping to her body, was

removed before testing the acupuncture points. The points for the liver and kidneys had a low electrical output, which signaled that these filters were still heavily involved in removing mercury. When the selenium tablet was placed on her skin, these points improved their electrical output. The selenium tablet was therefore able to provide much needed support to Angela's body while mercury was being eliminated. Perhaps the support of the selenium's magnetic field, which corrected the opposing field of mercury, had been instrumental in the lack of reaction to the previous treatment. More research is without doubt necessary in this area and well worth any allotted time if the health of the patient is to be improved as a result. Although the treatment was progressing slowly, there was an improvement in Angela's condition. Unfortunately though, she was unable to return to England for quite some time. For this reason, and to reduce the stress to her body further, she was tested for food sensitivity and found that tea, coffee, milk, wheat, beef, tomatoes and potatoes should be avoided.

This is a very strict diet, particularly as it was not possible to review the situation in a couple for week's time as would be normal. Angela was more than happy to try out this restricted diet because her condition had much improved. As with many people who complain of joint pain, the thoracic aortic plexus was burdened and milk sensitivity is usually identified when there is a problem with this plexus. Angela was no exception. As you will remember from Chapter 8, the thoracic aortic plexus is responsible for the blood supply to the upper body and tail of the pancreas that controls nucleoprotein metabolism and therefore uric acid, which results in pain and inflammation.

Nine kinds of amino acid are essential in our food, and a food that contains them all, is known as a complete protein food. Milk, eggs, cheese, meat, fish and lentils are such. Milk and its products provide very compact complete proteins necessary for basic bodybuilding and require the full complement of pancreatic enzymes for its proper digestion. If the full complement is not available due to malfunction, digestion is impaired. Perhaps this is why milk is the most common food to which people are allergic.

Very important here is the role of the adrenal glands, which were under pressure in Angela's case; it was difficult to elicit a response. The stresses of modern-day living can often be responsible for the overstimulation of the adrenal glands and, if we are not careful, the glands can be primed for action on a permanent basis. The surge of epinephrine (adrenaline) makes the heart beat faster and more strongly, this raises the blood pressure while at the same time constricting the blood vessels near the surface of the body and in the gut, redirecting the flow of blood towards the heart. Epinephrine is involved in the production of cortisone, which reduces inflammation, so the adrenal glands need to be functioning efficiently in any inflammatory condition. Often, changes to the focus of the eye, which Angela complained of, can indicate a malfunction of these glands. It was therefore most important for Angela to follow the guidelines below if she was to sustain her improvement. Angela returned home with a program of exercises, her chart for reflexology and many recipes to accommodate her new diet. She was also going to revisit her dentist with the purpose of establishing if a filling was indeed leaking.

Two weeks passed before Angela called. She was feeling isolated and rather upset about the whole situation that confronted her. A visit to her dentist had not proved fruitful: he refused to accept that a filling was leaking. Angela had paid regular visits to her dentist over many years and he felt insulted that a therapist from England was trying to tell him his job. Explaining that this was not the case, but that mercury could be the cause of her unexplained prolonged health problems, brought a torrent of abuse about scaremongering. This upset Angela, who didn't feel comfortable with the situation. As the treatments had improved her health upon returning home, Angela's husband encouraged her to find another dentist who was perhaps more sympathetic. After many enquiries, a dentist was discovered who was familiar with symptoms caused by amalgam. But before he would accept her as a patient, Angela had to fast for 2 days

and adhere to a 2-week diet so strict it was virtually impossible to achieve with a family to look after. I advised her to focus on her cleansing program and to continue the search for a more understanding dentist. Eventually a dentist was found who confirmed that a filling was indeed leaking. In fact, this dentist felt confident that there were at least five fillings that could fit this criterion. Unfortunately, I was not confident that Angela's body could cope with a removal at the present time and I advised her not to proceed with any replacement until her body was better prepared. This news can often be difficult for a patient to accept, especially when they start to feel better. Angela wanted to proceed as quickly as possible so she decided to visit the clinic.

FOURTH VISIT

During this visit, it was confirmed, after testing Angela's acupuncture points, that mercury was still the major toxin in her body – in particular in her liver and kidneys. However, they did respond to reflexology, which always improved the energy output. It is reassuring to know that support and self-help are readily available, but the reflexology must be sustained at home while these fillings are leaking. Angela was congratulated on the success of her home treatment program as her pancreas was less stressed; her exercises and diet were having an obvious effect. After careful consideration, it was decided that Angela was well enough to have one filling replaced, provided she coincided this with a visit to the clinic for assessment and she increased the frequency of her home treatment program to daily. The replacement substance that was available to Angela was ceramic. Alternative fillings are becoming more widespread; therefore research into material is increasing. Angela had one filling replaced and she arrived at the clinic 1 week after her dental visit.

As anticipated, the lymphatics were congested with mercury, silver, copper, nickel and anesthetic when her acupuncture points were tested. The anesthetic was obviously from the injection given by the dentist but it was the reason why Angela complained of a stiff neck and painful shoulders.

It wasn't until this stiff neck reappeared that she realized she had been free from this pain for weeks. Once a substance is identified in the lymphatics of the duodenum and jejunum there is usually marked discomfort in the neck region. As in previous cases this resulted in a malfunction of the energy to the abdominal muscles, which restricted the nerve supply to the upper spine and neck, and caused the pain. This will respond to Exercise 4 (the four-step exercise) and abdominal massage. If the offending substance is a recent introduction into the patient's environment then any congestion will usually respond to these exercises within a day or two.

Treatment

Full details of how to perform the exercises in the following list can be found in Appendix 1.

1. **Reflexology.** To the liver, kidneys, spleen, lungs, heart, adrenal glands, and lymph drainage points (see Fig. 10.2). Massage above and below the clavicles.
2. **Exercise 1, lymph cistern.**
3. **Red light exercise.**
4. **Abdominal massage.**
5. **Exercise 4, the four-step exercise.**
6. **Do-in.** Lightly tap over the whole of the chest and thyroid area then move down and do the same to either side of the lower rib cage.
7. **Reflexology.** To the liver, kidneys, spleen, heart, lungs, lymph drainage points followed by adrenal gland, large and small intestines, pancreas and lymph cistern. The homeopathic remedy Arnica was introduced.

Two days later, when Angela returned, her neck problem had almost disappeared and she was feeling none the worse for the episode. For this treatment session, the rowing boat exercise was included between steps 3 and 4. Holding a new set of charts for reflexology and the rowing boat exercise, she returned home to her family feeling more confident.

It was about 6 months before Angela returned again. She was feeling a little achy, but well. Because she had been feeling better she had decided to have some dental work done before her appointment with me, so another filling had been replaced. Following a similar procedure as on previous visits, her therapy went according to plan. Although there was evidence of amalgam in her system, lymphatic congestion would be minimal, providing she followed the strict program at home as before. Angela, however, was very frustrated about the amount of amalgam still in her mouth, particularly after reading reports of mercury causing depression, tiredness and bowel problems. The majority of her back teeth had been filled, many for more than 12 years. She was starting to feel so much better, particularly following a treatment, and she wanted to replace all her fillings and be done with it. The agitation she experienced was appreciated but the dangers were explained once more. After careful deliberation Angela agreed to be patient.

Three months later, Angela rang the clinic distraught: she had been diagnosed as suffering from polymyalgia rheumatica. This is an uncommon disease that is marked by pain and stiffness in the muscles of the hips, thighs, shoulders and neck. The cause is unknown, but it is thought to be associated with temporal arteritis or rheumatoid arthritis. Polymyalgia rheumatica affects twice as many women as men and is unusual before the age of 50. Symptoms can develop gradually or suddenly, making movement difficult. Morning stiffness is notable and often makes getting out of bed a problem. Weight loss and depression can also occur. The diagnosis, which is often difficult to confirm, is based on the patient's history, a physical examination and blood tests (including erythrocyte sedimentation rate (ESR)). The ESR is increased if the level of fibrinogen (a type of protein) in the blood is raised. Fibrinogen levels are usually found to be raised in response to inflammation, especially when caused by infection or an autoimmune disease (British Medical Association 1990: 416). So why did this suddenly happen to Angela?

As mentioned in Chapter 4, fibrinogen is capable of clotting while still in the body. The possibility of other substances, including mercury, adhering to this sticky mass and causing heavy congestion is very real. It is possible for the mass to stick to the walls of the lymphatic vessels, where it will distort electrical stimuli with its antagonistic magnetic field and prevent the free flow of messages through the tissues.

Angela was very upset, especially as she had great difficulty getting out of bed each morning, not to mention the many steps she had to negotiate in her home which was built into a hillside. Her knees in particular were very swollen and painful, and it was almost impossible to move her arms and shoulders. Small doses of corticosteroid drugs usually bring about an improvement in polymyalgia rheumatica within a few days. The dosage is gradually reduced and use of the drug can be discontinued within 2 years (British Medical Association 1990, p 816). Angela's doctor had prescribed cortisone for the inflammation but she was very reluctant to take this because of the side-effects. However, her condition was getting worse by the day. I suggested that she take the medication and discuss her concerns with her doctor. Angela rang the clinic a few days later, her sympathetic doctor had reassured her that he would monitor her blood and reduce the medication as soon as was feasible. It was during this conversation that Angela disclosed the fact that 4 weeks prior to the onset of her debilitating symptoms she had received two replacement fillings.

Apparently, she had chipped a tooth that the dentist had identified as leaking, and the dentist had suggested that she replace that filling and the adjacent one. Angela had agreed without thinking of the consequences. Her body would be totally congested with the debris from the fillings and this could well have contributed to the sudden onset of this condition.

Angela was given help over the telephone, by way of lymphatic clearance, but she didn't improve for more than a few hours at a time and a fifth visit was arranged.

FIFTH VISIT

When Angela arrived at the clinic she was very upset. The inflammation she was suffering was so bad it was not possible to touch any of her joints. The swelling and stiffness of the joints caused her immense pain and made getting on to the treatment couch almost impossible. On testing her acupuncture points, mercury was the most prevalent metal, with silver and nickel scattered in isolation. She responded to homeopathic remedies Belladonna and Ledum but she was still reluctant to take the cortisone because she was afraid of the lasting effects.

In general, metals are filtered out mainly by the liver through the bile ducts into the small intestine and out via the colon, whereas other items are filtered out by the nephrons in the kidneys and exit via the bladder. However, the kidneys do appear to take over from the liver (and vice versa) if either is overloaded with toxins. The pattern that emerged during investigation of metals leaving the body suggested right and left drift exit. This means that, once metals get into the bloodstream, they concentrate more on the right or left side of the body, and affect that side of the body more. They are filtered out by the right or left lobes of the liver and right or left kidney, respectively. Mercury is a left drift metal and will normally exit via the left lobe of the liver or, if this is overburdened, the left kidney. Angela showed evidence of mercury in both lobes of the liver and both kidneys. Silver is right drift and will therefore gravitate to the right exits. If these are highly congested – as Angela's were with mercury – the dominant metal (in Angela's case the silver) will sit in the body unable to find a way out. Intense reflexology of these zones is crucial and therefore dominated this treatment session.

SIXTH VISIT

Angela received treatment again 5 days later. The reflexology had indeed eased the congestion a little, her liver and kidneys appeared to be coping but her joints were still very badly affected by inflammation, although she assured me that the pain was not quite as bad. Belladonna tablets were taped to both knees, which would give local support and help with the inflammation. Angela returned home with a little more hope than when she arrived. I suggested that she take her doctor's advice regarding the cortisone, which would undoubtedly help with the inflammation.

Two weeks later Angela rang to say that she had discussed all aspects of her condition with her doctor and was now taking cortisone, her doctor had also prescribed Belladonna and Ledum to be administered intravenously.

SEVENTH VISIT

Ten weeks later, Angela returned to the clinic. The inflammation was no longer evident, she was walking much more easily, but mercury and silver were still present in her system. Cortisone was also identified in the initial bile ducts of her liver. This session consisted of reflexology and, because the inflammation had subsided, abdominal massage. The homeopathic remedies Belladonna and Ledum were still being effective and her body was responding to this combination. The selenium tablet that had been discarded prior to the fillings being removed was reintroduced and taped to her shoulder blades, but only for 2 days in every seven.

EIGHTH VISIT

Two days later Angela returned. The improvement was very obvious and good to witness. She was still very stiff in the mornings but some actions, like combing her hair, were more manageable. As inflammation was much reduced, massage to her neck and shoulders was possible, not only to ease the spasm in the muscles but also to relax a very tense patient. Breathing techniques were explained that would help to clear her system, to which she responded remarkably well. She made the journey home with mixed feelings. She was very frightened about the amalgam that was still present in her mouth and fretful that the condition that had descended upon her would escalate. Although there was a great deal of contact between myself and Angela, I didn't actually see her for 10 months. However, her progress had been remarkable in that time.

NINTH VISIT

The cortisone had been reduced but tests revealed that she no longer responded to

Belladonna and Ledum but to Hepar. Sulph. and Hammamelis. This was later reported to Angela's doctor, who was more than happy to cooperate in the combined treatments. The lymphatic drainage exercises became an important part of Angela's rehabilitation program, which she performed religiously at home.

Angela continued to improve. This was also reflected in the blood tests taken after each treatment, which allowed a steady reduction in the prescribed cortisone level. It has been 6 years since Angela was first diagnosed with polymyalgia rheumatica and her blood sedimentation levels were first recorded. It is interesting to note that, after each visit to England for a treatment, Angela's blood sedimentation reduced, on one such occasion (in March 1998) from 35 to 19 (Table 11.1).

There was one occasion, however, when Angela's doctor had to increase her cortisone following one of her many routine blood tests. Angela was not particularly aware of any alteration in her condition, so she was rather curious. Normally, severe joint pain and inflammation was an indication that the cortisone would have to be increased. What was very interesting was that 2 days prior to the blood test Angela had stubbed her toe, and was in a great deal of pain due to swelling and inflammation! Perhaps her toe, and not polymyalgia rheumatica, was the reason for the increased ESR level? The cortisone was duly reduced when the following blood test revealed the inflammation had subsided.

Table 11.1 Blood sedimentation results before and after treatments

Date	ESR level, and when taken
04.04.1995	20 before
12.05.1995	15 after
09.02.1996	18 before
13.03.1996	15 after
19.06.1996	30 before
30.10.1996	22 after
27.03.1998	33 before
17.04.1998	19 after
09.09.1998	21 before
26.10.1998	37 after

The careful removal of her fillings continued throughout this period, albeit very slowly. Both Angela and her dentist realized the importance of being patient and careful, so too did her doctor, who acknowledged the pattern of events after each filling had been removed. This resulted in a bout of pain and slight increase in inflammation, which was monitored carefully. Angela became adept in the management of the whole process of lymphatic drainage and is now quite confident and highly competent in all aspects of integrated therapy. Without home management of the therapy the situation could have had a totally different outcome.

TENTH VISIT

Angela was feeling particularly well when she arrived for this last treatment. The points for her liver and kidneys were also good, but there was still evidence of mercury in parts of her body. It was therefore decided to give deeper lymphatic drainage in the hope of eliminating entrenched mercury. Although Angela's blood sedimentation had increased on her return home, she had not felt a decline in her condition. This was probably due to her careful home management of the situation. Exercises 5 (bronchial plexus), 6 (brainstem) and 7 (lymph drainage of the heart) were introduced into this treatment program and are explained in the patient exercises in Appendix 2 (pp 180–182).

Angela visits every year, usually for her 'MOT'. Metals are still evident on occasions in her lymphatic system when her acupuncture points are tested. This is probably due to the years of constant infiltration and congestion caused by the leaking fillings. This will continue for some time yet, as the deeper lymphatics drain into the surface ones, so the need for caution still applies. Reflexology continues to support the organs and removal of toxic matter, which Angela is very capable of doing for herself. Her diet has been modified at each visit, making life much easier. Not only is she able to walk into town, but walking the dog twice a day is a pleasure. Angela's doctor has since confirmed that she is actually allergic to mercury. It is not surprising,

therefore, that her whole body rebelled when fillings were removed, overwhelming her lymphatic system and resonating an alien frequency that totally confused her whole body.

From experience gained over the years, amalgam should not be used in dental procedures. Amalgam containing mercury most certainly should not be removed without due care and attention and without careful consideration of the condition of the lymphatic system.

The data that are now available from many experts in this field, some of whom are quoted in this case history, should surely be considered further:

Mercury vapour measurements in the mouth before and after chewing gum for 10 minutes: *In the control group without fillings, the researchers were able to detect very small amounts of mercury vapour before chewing gum. After chewing gum for 10 minutes, the amount of mercury vapour measured remained the same. In the test group with amalgam fillings in their teeth, measurable amounts of mercury vapour were detected before they began chewing gum. After chewing gum for 10 minutes the researchers discovered a 15.5-fold increase in the amount of mercury vapour in their breath...It is thereby concluded that the possibility for significant mercury vapour exposure from dental amalgam in humans exists.* (Svare 1981)

Reporting on an international conference held in New York, dentist David Kennedy summarized:

It appears that mothers transfer mercury from their bloodstream to the unborn infant throughout pregnancy. We must reconsider whether we should place or remove fillings during pregnancy. All research shows that mercury is released into the blood during placement and removal of mercury fillings, there are some indications that mercury may be implicated in sudden infant death and other abnormalities. (Kennedy 1990)

A review by Sweden's Karolinska Institute (Martin 1990) states that:

Over time, mercury accumulates in organs, even when blood and urine tests show 'normal' levels, some mercury ends up in the brain. Dentists themselves have been found to have surprisingly large amounts of mercury in their pituitary glands.

In the UK, women are encouraged to visit their dentist when they are pregnant and any

treatment they receive is free of charge.
How many of these women had amalgam fillings replaced at this most vulnerable time?

The suggestion is not that amalgam fillings are wholly responsible for any form of arthritis, including polymyalgia rheumatica. Factors other than irresponsible removal of amalgam fillings could cause problems in people who do not have a lymphatic system that is functioning to its optimum efficiency. Unless there is evidence to support that existing fillings are leaking, they should remain in place if there is any doubt to the fitness of the person involved. When an amalgam filling is to be removed the following procedure is recommended and should be strictly adhered to.

The safe removal of amalgam fillings

Most dentists are extremely careful in the removal of amalgam fillings and cooperate in ensuring that the danger is minimized. To reduce the danger as far as possible, I recommend the following guidelines:

1. Practise breathing through your nose with your mouth open until you can do so without hesitation and for several minutes' duration.
2. Ask your dentist to allow you to sit in a semi-upright position during the removal process. The supine position will be quite all right once the removal process is finished.
3. The conscientious use of an aspirator, which sprays fine jets of water into the mouth and then sucks it out together with the bulk of metal detritus.
4. Do not hesitate to signal to your dentist the moment you feel that you have to swallow during the removal process, so that you can spit-out the debris instead of swallowing it.
5. After leaving the surgery, take a soft, damp, cotton handkerchief and carefully wipe out the dust. This could have accumulated on or under the tongue, on either side of the gums, and on the roof and back of the mouth. Use a new section of handkerchief for each part of the mouth.

There are many reasons given for not using ceramic fillings, mainly related to their durability. Dentists have been known to complain that they are unsuitable, particularly for back teeth, because they do not possess the strength of amalgam. However, many of my 'white' fillings are still in place after almost 15 years, but I do not use fluoride toothpaste. Fluorine attacks and oxidizes many metals and even glass. Fluorine is very evident in most dental procedures, including the dressings that are often packed into a cavity prior to filling.

Patient guide

Appendix 2 contains instructions to the patient on how to perform the exercises in the following list.

I would strongly advise any patient who is considering the removal of amalgam fillings unnecessarily to think again. However, if fillings are to be removed I would advise any patient to consult a therapist who is familiar with the dangers and to be guided by this person's expertise during the removal process to introduce each new step of the program when appropriate. Do not under any circumstances perform all of these steps at once until the lymphatic system is sufficiently adept in dealing with the toxic rubbish.

Self-help prior to the removal of an amalgam filling and after an amalgam filling has been removed, or if a leak is suspected prior to consultation involves:

Week one:

1. **Reflexology.** To the liver, kidneys, spleen, heart and lungs. Massage above and below the clavicle each night. Tape a selenium tablet between the shoulder blades for 1 week.
2. **The red light massage.**

If a filling has been removed, continue with the program as follows:

Week two:

1. **Reflexology.** To the liver, kidneys, spleen, heart, lungs and pancreas. Massage above and below the clavicle.
2. **The red light massage.**
3. **Abdominal massage.**
4. **Reflexology.** To the liver, kidneys, spleen, heart and lungs, and massage above and below the clavicle.

It would be advisable to repeat the program each evening for 2 weeks.

Week four:

   1. **Reflexology.** To the liver, kidneys, spleen, heart and lungs, and massage above and below the clavicle.
   2. **The red light massage.**
   3. **Abdominal massage.**
   4. **Exercise 1, lymph cistern.**
   5. **Red light massage.**
   6. **Abdominal massage.**
   7. **Do-in.** To the whole of the chest area. **The following exercises are only to be included at this stage providing your therapist is satisfied that your lymphatic system will accommodate their inclusion.** However, reflexology can be continued between each step if you so desire.
   8. **Exercise 4, the four-step exercise.**
   9. **Exercise 2, lungs and upper abdomen.**
   10. **Do-in.**
   11. **Exercise 5, bronchial plexus.** This is on the artery supplying the bronchi and bronchiole, and lies behind the sternum on the 3rd sternal groove. Stimulation of this plexus is achieved by clearing the lymphatics behind the sternum using a simple massage.
   12. **Exercise 6, brainstem.** The therapist will be familiar with the massage technique that is required.
   13. **Exercise 7, lymph drainage of the heart.** This exercise should be performed only after Exercises 2, 5 and 6, and *never* on its own.
   14. **Reflexology.** To the liver, kidneys, spleen, heart, lungs and lymph drainage points, and massage above and below the clavicles. Followed by reflexology to the thyroid gland, adrenal gland, large and small intestines, pancreas, lymph cistern, lungs and heart, and finishing with the liver, kidneys, spleen, heart and lungs (see Fig. 11.1, pp 100–101).

The reflexology steps should be completed in a total of 15 minutes. Once an improvement has been achieved, the program need only be completed once a week or as directed by the therapist.

Supplements[3]

- Vitamin B1 (thiamin): helps to support the pancreas once the nerve supply has been corrected and relieves pain and stiffness in the joints.
- Vitamin B3 (niacin): appears to help cortisone (if it is being taken) penetrate to the necessary areas of inflammation.
- Vitamin C: can help the adrenal gland to produce cortisone and also help with inflammation. Take 2 g a day (check with your doctor or therapist first).
- New Era tissue salts, calcium fluoride and magnesium phosphate: for inflammation and to relieve pain.
- Celery seed: is very useful for acidic conditions such as arthritis, gout, rheumatism and lumbago.
- Arnica and Belladonna homeopathic remedies have helped many patients with arthritic conditions.
- Vitamin E: 400–600 iu per day as an antioxidant.
- Extra virgin olive oil: 1 tablespoon each morning, $\frac{1}{2}$ hour before breakfast can be beneficial, especially for stiff joints and to assist bowel movements.
- Ginseng: raises the energy in the pancreas.
- Selenium ACE: can be beneficial in the removal of amalgam from the body after all the fillings have been replaced.
- Magnesium: as a supplement. Without magnesium, calcium cannot be absorbed. It appears that magnesium stimulates calcitonin, a hormone that increases calcium in the bones. Magnesium is believed to prevent calcium formation in the tissues, so it is beneficial as a first aid to help prevent calcium spur from forming around joints.
- Massage oil: add five drops of essential oil of ginger to 10 ml castor oil; although sticky, this will help stiff joints and muscles.
- Have a diet rich in fish and chicken, avoid red meat if possible.

Patients sometimes complain of a rapid heartbeat after an anesthetic administered by

---

[3] Not all of these supplements should be taken at once.

their dentist. I would recommend Citanest anesthetic 3% or 4% Octapressin, which your dentist will possibly be using anyway, but it might be wise to check first.

The reflexology charts and acupuncture points that are relevant for this case study are shown in Figs 11.1 and 11.2 and are to be used in conjunction with ISR in association with the particular lymphatic drainage techniques for integrated therapy.

REFERENCES

British Medical Association 1990 Complete family health encyclopaedia. Dorling Kindersley, London

Daily Mail, September 10, 1990

Egglestone D W 1984 Mercury fillings suppress the immune system. Journal of Prosthetic Dentistry; 51(5): 617–623

Horton C (ed) 1985 Atlas of anatomy. Marshall Cavendish, London

Martin S 1990 Mercury, the toxic time-bomb in your teeth. Here's Health; June: 18–20

Oschman J 2000 Energy medicine. Harcourt Publishers, London

Pickering Pick T, Howden R 1988 Gray's Anatomy (Classic Collector's edition). Crown Publishers, UK

Svare 1981 Journal of Dental Research; 60: 35, 39

Voll R 1984 The 850 EAV measurement points of the meridians and vessels including the secondary vessels. Medizinisch Literarische Verlagsgesellschaft mbH, Uelzen

Ziff S 1984 The toxic time bomb. Aurora Press, London

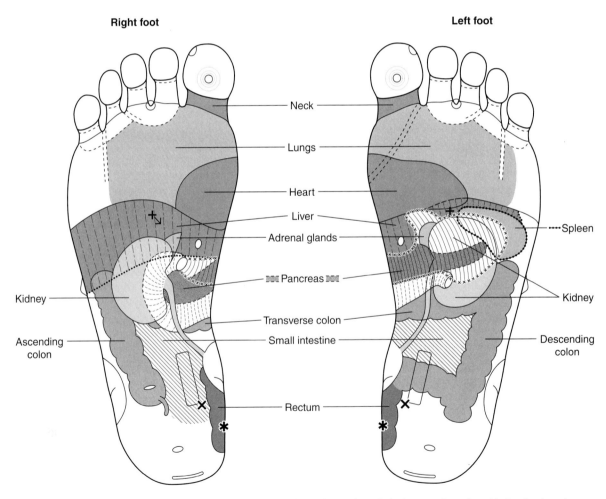

Figure 11.1   Reflexology chart for the liver, kidneys, spleen, heart, lungs, lymph drainage points, thyroid gland, adrenal gland, large and small intestines and pancreas. © F. Fox, used with permission.

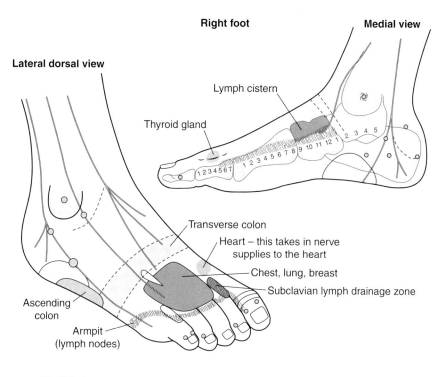

Right foot

Medial view

Lateral dorsal view

Lymph cistern

Thyroid gland

Transverse colon

Heart – this takes in nerve
supplies to the heart

Chest, lung, breast

Subclavian lymph drainage zone

Ascending
colon

Armpit
(lymph nodes)

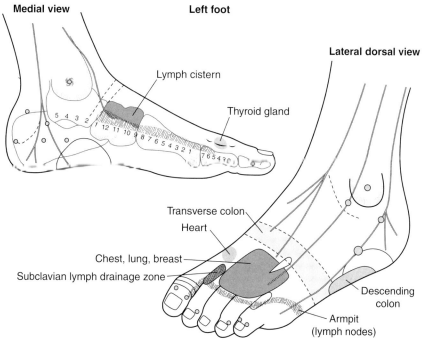

Medial view

Left foot

Lateral dorsal view

Lymph cistern

Thyroid gland

Transverse colon

Heart

Chest, lung, breast

Subclavian lymph drainage zone

Descending
colon

Armpit
(lymph nodes)

Figure 11.1   (*continued*).

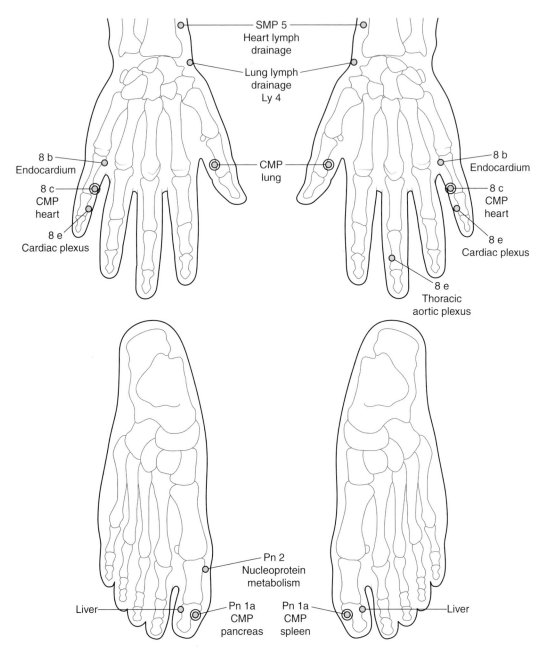

Figure 11.2 Relevant acupuncture points. The points illustrated are for fingertip testing, assessment, and acupressure only. CMP, control measurement point; SMP, summation measurement point.

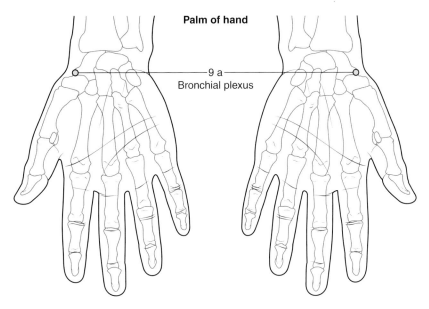

Figure 11.2   (*continued*).

12

Asthma

CHILDHOOD ASTHMA

FIRST VISIT

James, a little boy of five, was a chronic asthma sufferer. As the eldest of four children he was very bright, with a sense of responsibility towards his younger brothers and sister beyond his years. Bronchodilators helped him to breathe and James's condition, which required him to be hospitalized with increasing frequency, meant that he was missing a considerable amount of schooling.

The consultants looking after James had informed the family that the strength of medication required at the moment to control his symptoms was quite high for one so young. James's condition was indeed getting worse and the attacks had increased in frequency over the last 8 months. After hospitalization, James's breathing was usually quite good for a couple of months, but then the attacks started again. A hereditary factor often plays a part in a child's susceptibility to developing the condition and James's paternal grandfather did suffer from asthma.

The lungs are a mass of airways, the largest of which are the bronchi, which divide off from the trachea to the left and right, each entering its respective lung, where they branch out into the smaller tubes called bronchioles that end in air sacs called alveoli. Awake or asleep, we breathe an average of 12 times a minute and breathe in and out more than 8000 liters of air during any 24 hours.

Asthma is a partial obstruction of the bronchi and bronchioles caused by inflammation. The condition usually begins in childhood and can be caused by an allergic reaction. Medical allergy tests can reveal house dust, house dust mite, pollens and animal fur as the triggers. Medication similar to the type that James was prescribed is commonplace in asthma sufferers. These drugs, which help to settle the inflammation and open the airways, are usually taken on a daily basis, some as a preventive.

On testing James's acupuncture points, all the lung points – intestines, liver, kidneys, brainstem and bronchial and mediastianal plexus – were congested with benzoate, which is a preservative, and methane gas. James was found to be sensitive to cows milk, potatoes and white flour. Other substances to which he was sensitive were benzoate and the brand of soap powder that his mother was using.

Benzoates (E210–219) are a group of preservatives produced from benzoic acid and used in many fats, vegetable lard and oil, soft drinks and diet drinks; they are to be found in many of the drinks that children enjoy. They also occur in various perfumes, soaps, cosmetics, cough mixtures and other medications.

Synonyms include: benzoic acid; sodium salt; benzoate of soda; sodium benzoic acid; and Antimol.

From the point of view of providing safe food, preservatives that prevent the growth of microorganisms would appear to be more beneficial than moldy food. However, many of the preservatives used can have adverse effects on some people and have been known to cause irritation to the respiratory tract (coughing and shortness of breath), the gastrointestinal tract, the skin and the eye.

James was always thirsty and drank copious amounts of fizzy drinks that had sodium benzoate as one of the ingredients.

Benzyl alcohol, another derivative of benzoic acid, has been linked to neonatal cardiovascular collapse – dubbed 'gasping baby syndrome'. This was established after a series of new-borns died or developed a severe respiratory illness associated with gasping metabolic acidosis (an overly acidic body pH) and blood abnormalities. The cause of this syndrome was eventually determined to be intravenous flush solutions and medications containing benzyl alcohol. The incidence of premature infant mortality, intraventricular haemorrhage and severe neurological symptoms reduced significantly after discontinuation of the use of benzyl alcohol in intravenous drugs proposed for infants. (Thomas 2001)

Pesticides

On 13 January 2000, S.C. Johnson, an American manufacturer of pesticide products, advised retail stores across the country to remove from their shelves the products 'AllerCare, the Dust Mite Carpet Powder' and 'AllerCare, the Dust Mite Allergen Spray', after complaints from people with severe allergies and asthma. Reports came via a help-line that reactions included asthma attacks, respiratory problems, burning sensations and skin irritation. In most cases, the reported effects began within 15–30 minutes of using the product(s). In addition, the US Environmental Protection Agency received reports of reactions in some pets. Both these products contain the active ingredient benzyl benzoate.

Milk

Dr Jonathan Wright, a nutritional pioneer, finds that the 'vast majority of cases of childhood asthma are of a "gastrointestinal origin", that is, children with asthma tend to have poor stomach acid. In one study of 200 children in 1931, four out of five were found to have low stomach acid' (Wright 1996). Although food allergy often causes this stomach acid problem, one of the big culprits is cows milk. In 1979 a researcher called Kokkonen, who examined stomach acid in children before and after giving them milk, discovered that even a single dose of cows milk destroyed the stomach lining in sensitive children. Afterwards, the gastric acid levels in these children were one-third those of a normal group. Kokkonen (1996) also found that the children's stomachs took up to 6 months to recover from this one dose – and that was with complete avoidance of all dairy products and any other allergens.

Gas

The main source of heating for James's family was from a gas fire. The gas cooker often supplemented the heating when it was very cold as the family ate in the kitchen. Natural gas is promoted as the 'clean fuel'. This might be so from the point of view of visible or smog-producing residues, but for the chemically susceptible person gas can be the worst form of fuel. Most cities in the early part of this century were supplied with artificial gas derived from coal. With the completion of a national gas line network after the Second World War, most cities switched to natural gas. However, from the point of view of chronic disease, whether the gas is artificial or natural does not matter, as both can cause problems for those with the chemical sensitivity. Natural gas is delivered at much higher pressures than the artificial product, and this can cause a serious problem of leakage if the pipes were originally constructed for the transmission of artificial gas. Gas, being lighter than air, tends to rise from the kitchen into the rest of the house. The greater the amount of piping and the number of outlets, from pilots and other automatic devices on gas appliances, the greater will be the probability of leaks.

One of the most amazing features of this gas problem is the incredible sensitivity of some people to its presence. Simply shutting off a gas appliance is not enough. In many circumstances, the gas appliance must be completely removed from the premises if a person is affected by gas in a bad way. For the seriously ill there is no substitute for complete removal of the offending appliance. This is because even a non-working appliance continues to give off odor from the gas that it has absorbed over the years. In many cases, when a cooker was removed for the benefit of one member of the family, other members of that family also reported an improvement in health. A gas cooker was removed from the home of one patient, a girl with persistent headaches. Her mother, who was not a patient, reported an unsuspected benefit. While cooking with gas, she had often become highly irritable. She would scream at anyone who came into her kitchen. As she frequently had a kitchen knife in her hand when she started screaming, this created a bad atmosphere at dinnertime. With the removal of the gas cooker, her temper tantrums quickly subsided. What had appeared to be a potential 'psychological problem' was solved simply by removing a hidden environmental pollutant (Randolph & Moss 1980).

The management of asthma and other respiratory conditions

With breathing problems such as bronchitis, asthma and emphysema, the bronchial and mediastinal plexuses are usually disturbed by very congested lymphatics nearby. The bronchial nodes are scattered over the surface of the bronchi and are to be found where the bronchi divides and even extend to the bronchioles. These nodes drain upwards toward the subclavian veins and are also responsible for draining lung tissue. It is thought the mediastinal nodes either empty separately or join the mammary ducts to empty into the subclavian veins. The mediastinum contains the heart, trachea, esophagus, thymus gland, the major blood vessels entering and leaving the heart, lymph nodes, lymphatic vessels and nerves

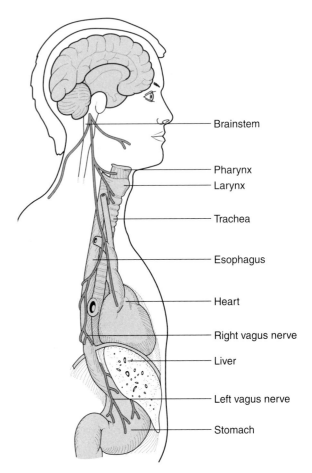

Figure 12.1 The vagus nerve.

(including the vagus nerve and phrenic nerves) (British Medical Association 1990, p 668). For this reason, any distortion from congested lymphatics to the mediastinal and bronchial plexuses should be kept to a minimum. The contour of the chest wall is significant in asthmatics, particularly those who are flat-chested with sagging ribs, and lack of tone in the muscles, which prevents circulation and tissue tone of the lung, is a result of this distortion of energy. The lymph drainage exercises that are outlined later in the chapter will help to correct these malfunctioning intercommunications and allow the nourishment of tissues to be re-established.

The vagus nerve is the longest of the cranial nerves and branches extensively (Fig. 12.1). From the brainstem at the back of the neck,

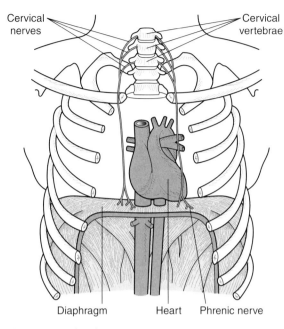

Figure 12.2 The phrenic nerves.

through the neck and chest to the abdomen, it has branches to most of the major organs in the body, including the lungs, heart and much of the digestive system. It wields its effects on target organs by releasing the chemical acetylcholine, which causes a narrowing of the bronchi and slowing of the heart rate. Acetylcholine also stimulates the production of stomach acid and pancreatic juice, stimulates the activity of the gall bladder and increases peristalsis of the digestive tract. Branches of the vagus nerve supply the muscles of the larynx and trachea and are therefore involved in the actions of swallowing, coughing and sneezing, and in speech quality (British Medical Association 1990, p 1043).

The phrenic nerves emerge from the third, fourth and fifth cervical nerves in the neck (Fig. 12.2). Passing down through the chest on each side of the diaphragm they carry impulses to and from the diaphragm and play an important part in controlling breathing from nervous system instruction to either contract or relax. This is a long journey from the neck down to the bottom of the chest and injury or distortion of energy to one of these nerves could result in a part of the diaphragm being paralysed (British Medical Association 1990, p 802).

The vagus and phrenic nerves play a vital role in the management of asthma and any other condition associated with the respiratory system. The functions of these nerves are reliant on their electrical impulses finding their target organs. Every function of the nervous system is the result of the activities of neurons and their interconnectivity. Similarly, oscillation of the heart's electrical activity is not confined to the heart muscle but is propagated through the vascular system, perivascular connective tissue and living matrix to all parts of the body (Oschman 2000, p 95). When all of the body's communication channels are open, this interconnectivity is possible but is only achievable if the lymphatic system is able to do its job of elimination effectively, thereby removing any interference within the range of the magnetic fields and signals.

Lymph drainage of the lungs is of paramount importance when dealing with such problems as asthma, bronchitis or edema. Overloading of the lung lymphatic usually has a detrimental effect on the deep acupuncture meridians of the colon, which link the superficial meridians in the front of the shoulders to the transverse colon, right and left. Clearing the lymph nodes under the intercostal spaces both in front and in the back of the rib cage can be achieved by do-in (see Appendix 2, Fig. A2.3). As soon as the congestion is cleared, a distinct growl in the abdomen can be heard as the colon reacts to the sudden influx of extra energy via the deep meridian. This relationship between the lung and colon is of course well recognized by acupuncture practitioners. It is, however, another reminder of the interconnecting energy fields that exist within the body. It has become evident in severe cases of asthma, bronchitis or severely overloaded lung lymphatics that the endocardium of the heart, both right and left, can become burdened. This can easily be checked on acupuncture points (Ht 8b) on the base of the little finger. Signs and symptoms of congestion of the endocardium are low or high blood pressure, pallor, rapid pulse, dizziness or even fainting. Do-in at the bottom of the sternum is usually very successful in clearing this fault.

Asthma is reaching epidemic proportions in Western countries. In the UK, over 10% of all prescription costs are related to asthma patients, with over 4% of the adult population and 6% of all children needing frequent medical supervision. Conventional treatment appears to focus almost exclusively on steroid medicines taken by way of inhalers. However, new research is revealing that some of the answers in the effective prevention and treatment of this illness might lie with the food that is eaten.

Asthma is a serious condition and must be treated accordingly. However, many people might actually be suffering from a combination of food or chemical sensitivity with lymphatic congestion.

Treatment

First and foremost, any substances that may trigger a response had to be removed from James's diet. He was therefore only given pure fruit juice, with water added. There are proprietary brands of fizzy drinks available without benzoate, but these are usually more expensive. I advised James's mother that, whenever she was cooking with gas, there should always be plenty of ventilation in the kitchen – whatever the weather a door or window should be open, for the benefit of everyone concerned, not only James. If a gas fire is burning in the main living room it is preferable not to sit directly in front of it but to the side and have the room ventilated. Many patients, especially elderly patients, attending for treatments have shown lymphatics heavily contaminated by gas and, when questioned, all have invariably spent many hours sitting in front of the gas fire without ventilation. Patients who have changed to alternative forms of heating have all reported improvements to their breathing problems. For those patients who have no choice other than gas for heating it would be advisable to ventilate their bedrooms adequately, and patients who suffer from any breathing problems should if possible try to reduce the amount of gas appliances in the home. Portable gas heaters can have similar consequences: one patient, a shop owner was suffering irritation to the nose and throat, and sinusitis, with the resulting mucus draining down the windpipe at night. When her portable gas heater was removed and her lymphatics were drained, all of her symptoms disappeared.

The patient should follow the program only for reflexology each evening for about 15 minutes.

Appendix 2 contains instructions to the patient on how to perform the exercises in the following list.

1. **Reflexology.** To the liver, kidneys, spleen, lungs and lymph drainage points followed by massage above and below the clavicles (see Fig. 12.3, pp 116–117). The technique was demonstrated to James's mother and the importance of these areas being massaged each evening was stressed.
2. **The red light massage.**
3. **Exercise 1, lymph cistern.** This exercise should be done twice.
4. **Do-in.** Gently to the base of the sternum for at least 3 minutes.
5. **Reflexology.** To the liver, kidneys, spleen, lungs and heart (see Fig. 12.3, pp 116–117) with massage above and below the clavicles.

SECOND VISIT

One week later James's mother reported an improvement in James's breathing, although he was still very wheezy. This second treatment session followed much the same lines as the previous one but with the inclusion of back massage concentrating on the occiput. It is here that the vagus nerve emerges from the brainstem and can often be impeded by a spasm in the muscle on either or both sides of the neck, where it meets with the occipital ridge. Massage to the cervical ganglia, including the whole neck area, needs intense concentration, particularly the path taken by the vagus nerves before they travel down the body. This time, the treatment program to follow at home included abdominal massage.

1. **Reflexology.** To the liver, kidneys, spleen, lungs, lymph drainage points (see Fig. 12.3, pp 116–117) and massage above and below the clavicles.

2. **The red light massage.**

3. **Exercise 1, lymph cistern.** Do this exercise twice.

4. **Do-in.** Gently to the base of the sternum for at least 3 minutes.

5. **Abdominal massage.** This was demonstrated to James's mother.

6. **Do-in.** Gently to the base of the sternum for at least 3 minutes.

7. **Reflexology.** To the liver, kidneys, spleen, lungs and heart, with massage above and below the clavicles. Followed by reflexology to the lymph cistern, small and large intestines, and hypothalamus (see Fig. 12.3, pp 116–117). The final reflexology massage should take about 15 minutes in total to complete. Reflexology should continue nightly and the exercise steps should be included twice a week for 4 weeks.

THIRD VISIT

James's mother reported a happier child. His sleep had been less disturbed and he didn't appear to be as wheezy. This treatment session was the same as the last. The exercise and reflexology program continued at home for a further two weeks.

FOURTH VISIT

Success of the previous treatment enabled the inclusion of other steps at this treatment session: Exercises 2 (lungs and upper abdomen), 5 (bronchial plexus) and 6 (the brainstem), with do-in in between each exercise:

1. **Reflexology.** To the liver, kidneys, spleen, lungs, heart and lymph drainage points (see Fig. 12.3, pp 116–117) followed by massage above and below the clavicles.

2. **Exercise 1, lymph cistern.** Should be done twice.

3. **Do-in.** Gently to the base of the sternum for at least 3 minutes.

4. **Exercise 2, lungs and upper abdomen.** To clear the lungs and upper abdomen. James had difficulty mastering this exercise so I introduced do-in to clear the lymph nodes under

the intercostal spaces both in the front and to the back of the rib cage. These areas should be tapped lightly for a total of 3 minutes.

5. **Do-in.** To the base of the sternum.

6. **Exercise 5, bronchial plexus.**

7. **Do-in.** To the base of the sternum.

8. **Exercise 6, the brainstem.**

9. **Repeat Exercise 1, lymph cistern.**

10. **Do-in.** To the base of the sternum.

It is vital to remember that those patients who have to continue using their medication can suffer filters that are permanently trying to clear. The amount of lymphatic drainage must reflect this and be aptly apportioned. It is necessary at this stage in the program for the therapist to monitor the areas of congestion and instruct the patient on those steps that are to form part of the self-help program. Do not be hasty and introduce new steps into the program of a patient who is obviously very ill; it is more advantageous to proceed slowly. This will prevent clogging of the all-important filters, enhance results and prevent any adverse reaction to this cleansing program.

11. **Reflexology.** To the liver, kidneys, spleen, lungs, heart and lymph drainage points with massage above and below the clavicles, followed by reflexology to the lymph cistern, small and large intestines, and hypothalamus (see Fig. 12.3, pp 116–117). The final reflexology massage should take about 15 minutes in total to complete. Reflexology should continue nightly and include the exercise steps once a week for 2 weeks if the patient is progressing well through the therapy sessions.

The patient must drink eight glasses of water a day for 3 days after following a treatment program.

FIFTH VISIT

James ran into my treatment room to greet me 2 weeks later. However, his mother felt that the last treatment had not been as successful as previous ones; James apparently appeared to be more tired than usual. On testing the acupuncture points they were all congested but the filters were clear. This treatment was identical to the previous one, with the inclusion of Exercise 7 (lymph drainage of the heart).

    1. **Reflexology.** To the liver, kidneys, spleen, lungs, heart, lymph drainage points and massage above and below the clavicles.
    2. **Exercise 1, lymph cistern.**
    3. **The red light massage.** Every day.
    4. **Do-in.** To the bottom of the sternum.
    5. **Abdominal massage.**
    6. **Do-in.**
    7. **Exercise 2, lungs and upper abdomen.**
This exercise was introduced here to clear the congestion to James's mediastinal plexus.

An alternative to exercise 2, especially for young children, is do-in to clear the lymph nodes under the intercostal spaces both in the front and to the back of the rib cage. Tapping gently, move up and down the rib cage, back and front. Clearance of the lungs and heart can be checked on NS 2 on the epicondyle at the base of the index finger lateral side.
    The bronchial plexus, which is on the artery supplying the bronchi and bronchiole, lies behind the sternum on the 3rd sternal groove. Stimulation of this plexus is achieved by clearing the lymphatics behind the sternum by massage. Exercise 5 (bronchial plexus) does this job superbly.

    8. **Exercise 5, bronchial plexus.**
    9. **Do-in.** To the bottom of the sternum.
    10. **Exercise 6, the brainstem.**
    11. **Do-in.** To the bottom of the sternum.
    12. **Exercise 7, lymph drainage of the heart.** This exercise should be performed only after exercises 2, 5 and 6, and never on its own.
    13. **Repeat Exercise 1, lymph cistern.**
    14. **Do-in.** To the base of the sternum for a total of 3 minutes.
    15. **Reflexology.** To the liver, kidneys, spleen, lungs, heart, lymph drainage points, sides and back of the neck. Massage above and below the clavicles, followed by lymph cistern, and reflexology to the intestines and hypothalamus. Finish the sequence with the liver, kidneys, spleen and lungs (see Fig. 12.3, pp 116–117).

The patient should be encouraged to alternate these exercises once a week but reflexology to the above zones should be carried out each evening until the condition becomes more manageable.
    During this time of cleansing, the patient should drink as much water as possible.

SIXTH VISIT

This visit brought with it much discussion. James had suffered from bouts of eczema. The condition was not too distressing and it was assumed that it was related to his asthma. However, it cleared completely within 5 days of the last treatment. The wheezing had greatly subsided and disturbed nights were less frequent. The most revealing disclosure was in James's manner. He had become extremely calm, a side to his character that had never previously been revealed.
    Subsequent treatments identified chlorine in James's system. This ongoing cleansing is so important for an asthmatic. Any irritant or contact with an allergic substance can happen at any time and trigger an attack. However, if the lymphatics are maintaining their cleansing process then the immune system will be improving in efficiency. This expected improvement would be of benefit in reducing the recovery time from subsequent asthmatic attacks or even to reduce the rate of occurrence. As the deeper lymphatics become more mobile, the emerging material might have been contained within the vessels for quite a considerable time and be the original cause of any physiological fault. For this reason they must be identified as they surface, in the hope that they too can be removed from the patient's environment. The body's communication channels and interconnecting energy fields will undoubtedly be challenged again and again as the lymphatics clear and must be balanced accordingly. Prolonged disturbance of vital energy could result in permanent damage. For this reason early detection of physiological faults that could result in asthma should be the focus of discussion and research, particularly as this

condition, as reported is reaching epidemic proportions.

Chlorine is found in some medications, toothpastes and soap powders, antiseptics, disinfectants, swimming pools and sterilization substances that are used for baby's bottles. The latter are convenient for busy mums, but a possible health risk for babies. All substances that the baby may come into contact with, including formulas, can be checked for their suitability by using ISR.

Sodium hypochlorite and Sodium dichlorisocyanurate are found in sterilizing solutions for baby's bottles (see Further Reading). There are reports that these two solutions do not *off*gas (discharge of vapor into the atmosphere) and are relatively harmless, but the safest alternative to any chemical is a sterilizing unit that emits steam. Purified water can be used for this purpose, or water can be left standing for approximately 45–60 minutes to allow the chlorine to evaporate.

James continued to improve, although there were a few setbacks along the way, usually when he didn't control his diet through lack of family funds. His GP was impressed with the improvement and progress, especially as no further increase in potency of the medication was needed. James didn't need to use his inhalers as frequently now, and this situation was carefully monitored by his family and his GP.

Note: All asthmatics should carry their medication with them at all times, regardless of the improvement in their condition. They might be exposed to an irritant without their knowledge, and this could trigger an attack. It must be stressed again that asthmatics should not attempt all of the lymph drainage exercises in one go, or following a prolonged break in the program. Lymphatic hygiene of the type promoted in the program for James should ideally be part of a weekly routine. In this way any irritant that might have been absorbed can quickly be eliminated.

James's mother must be congratulated for her total involvement in the treatment program. She scanned all foods and drinks for their contents, as well as soaps and shampoos (many baby shampoos also contain benzoate or other

chemicals and much diligence is needed in rooting them out). However, the scanning of all substances, including food and toiletries, for their suitability for any child can be ascertained with the help of ISR and a surrogate.

Benzoate has been identified in the lymphatics and nerve plexuses of many children who have suffered from sleep and behavior problems, asthma and headaches. Chlorine can usually be identified in the lymphatics of patients with breathing problems.

ADULT ASTHMA

Sheila, a woman of 45, was diagnosed as asthmatic when she was 6 years of age, shortly after recovering from a childhood disease. Her medication of bronchodilators was similar to those used by James and was administered each day as a preventive measure. She was also having treatment for an underactive thyroid, in the form of thyroxine. Sheila was a nurse and very competent in all aspects of treatment and management of asthma. Testing her acupuncture points showed she was very congested with sulfur and chlorine. These substances can often be found in medication. Sulfur can also be found in antidandruff shampoo, some herbal shampoos, dried fruit, ginger, garlic, and medicines and cream preparations for the treatment of acne.

Chlorine in the lymphatics is often the result of using too much soap powder, but can come from other sources, including medication and tap water, to which we are constantly exposed.

An article from *What doctors don't tell you* (2001) on additives in medication makes very interesting reading:

Some individuals dependent on inhalers and other breathing aids develop paradoxical bronchospasm after they inhale their medication. In the past, such reactions were attributed to the presence of sulfites. However, these have been removed in some preparations and been replaced with benzalkonium chloride and chlorofluorocarbons to name but a few. In some asthmatic patients, benzalkonium chloride can produce significant respiratory distress. In a study by Zhang and colleagues of 28 asthmatics, a significant decrease in lung function – which began within a minute and lasted up to 60 minutes – was observed after benzalkonium chloride administration.

Sheila's areas of congestion were similar to those of James, with the inclusion of the cardiac ganglion.

The cardiac ganglion is located on the arch of the aorta. Any congestion of, or disturbance from, lymphatic stasis to this ganglion appears to contribute to arrhythmia. Lymph spaces are found almost everywhere and must be considered if we want to have healthy tissues. Whenever there is muscle inflexibility or strain we will find the lymph spaces, vessels and nodes more or less blocked by undue tension and altered vascularization. The lymph flow must move continually onwards, just like the venous blood, or there will be pathological changes as a result of the inactivity. The lymph passes through nodes continuously in a normal tissue condition. The arrest of this flow, through any of the causes that obstruct the activities of the nodes or the conveying properties of the lymph vessels, will mean a changed lymph substance. If the nodes collect and retain lymph laden with toxic products, suppuration will result. If this occurs in the bronchial nodes, there is danger of infection in the lung tissue from the broken-down nodes that lie along the branches of the bronchial tubes.

The lymph spaces between the bundles of cardiac muscles in the connective tissue connect with the vessels in the endocardium and epicardium. Vasomotor instability of the coronary arteries and blood vessels leaving the heart supply to the various cardiac nerves and plexuses can cause a change in the lymph spaces which, in time will produce a cardiac variation of rhythm (Millard 1922). 'This altered rhythm and lymphatic congestion may also weaken one or more valves of the heart' (Fox, unpublished). The cardiac nerve runs down the neck behind the common carotid artery. It lies upon the longus colli muscle and crosses in front of the inferior thyroid artery. Filaments from the cardiac nerves communicate with the thyroid branches from the middle cervical ganglion.

On examination of Sheila's neck, lymphatic congestion of the nodes in the midline and also

at the root of the neck in the triangular interval between the clavicle, the sternomastoid and the trapezius muscles was found. Whenever there is congestion in this area of the neck, identified by the tightness of the muscles and hard lymph nodes it usually signifies malfunctioning muscles of the diaphragm and/or thyroid instability. A number of patients medically diagnosed with heart conditions all exhibited hard tight muscles in this area of the neck. Exercise 10 (thyroid and parathyroid lymph nodes) and the red light massage (see Appendix 1) will help to reduce any spasm that might have formed here and encourage sluggish lymph nodes to drain into the drainage points. This can take some time and requires patience not only from the patient, who works on the drainage exercises at home, but from the therapist also. This very effective massage will eventually encourage energetic interactions between all of the nerves in this area. However, it could be 3 weeks before you can identify correct stimuli from the plexuses.

Patients who suffer from high blood pressure could also suffer a spasm in the triangular interval area. A spasm regularly forms in the longus colli muscles. This generally has an influence on the muscles either side of the cervical vertebrae, which can become almost rigid. However, Exercise 6 (the brainstem) will usually be effective in this instance, together with the red light massage.

Sheila's points for the hypothalamus were registering a low energy, which can be a common occurrence with asthmatics. A focus here could mean that some substance is trapped in one or more capillary beds within its wall, depriving it of the blood supply necessary to function normally. As an autonomic nervous system regulator, not only the lungs but also the diaphragm is dependent upon proper signals from the hypothalamus to allow the web of muscle fibers connected to the lower six ribs to contract and flatten during breathing. Lack of rib movement could be due to rigid costal muscles where lymph flow is checked from the intercostal vessel and nodes. There must be freedom of chest movement if we are to expect free lymph flow and improved breathing. The lymphatics that drain the back and front of the chest (organ 1d and 2) on the medial side of the fourth finger of the right hand will give a good indication of congestion. However, toxic matter can sometimes pass from these lymphatics into the lung nodes (check the right lung drainage Ly 4) located in the intercostal spaces 6 and 7 on the side of the rib cage.

The muscles of Sheila's diaphragm were obviously not receiving the correct impulses because they were extremely taut. In fact, the whole area felt like a solid ball, which explained why she was unable to breathe correctly.

Treatment

This first treatment varied very little from that of James, except that attention was also directed towards the taut muscles of the diaphragm. Please note that after the last breathing exercise but before reflexology, gentle massage below the sternum is required. As the muscles relax under your fingers you might feel inclined to increase the depth of the massage.

SECOND VISIT

Three weeks later Sheila returned and was delighted that she had barely had to use her inhalers since the last visit. The nerve impulses that had been obscured due to taut muscles were now allowed to connect with vital organs. This reflected the speed with which Sheila progressed. In a matter of weeks more steps were introduced into her treatment program, with equal success. The treatment program was identical to that of James except that results were very much quicker and included Exercise 10 (thyroid and parathyroid lymph nodes).

Often, bronchial infection and enlarged nodes in the mediastinal area will be reflected upon the drainage of the esophagus as the lymph is collected into these nodes before it is dispatched into the thoracic duct. Congestion of lymph, however, can occur in any of the nodes that lie adjacent to the esophagus and the exits of the drainage points (identified by edema or nodular enlargement above the clavicles) preventing the

lymph from being discharged and this pressure is likely to affect the thyroid gland.

Exercise 10: Thyroid and parathyroid lymph nodes

1. Massage deep into the tissues above and below the clavicle several times, spending some time on the lymph drainage points.

2. Massage deep into the acromioclavical joint (at the shoulder joint).

3. The red light massage should follow.

4. With the thumb and forefinger of the left hand, massage down either side of the larynx and out along the clavicles, above and below. Do exactly the same with the other hand. The patient under the guidance of the therapist best performs this exercise. See Appendix 2, p 183.

THIRD VISIT

Three weeks later Sheila returned, having been to her doctor to report what she described as little short of a miracle. Not only had she dispensed with her inhalers but most of the aching joints she attributed to her work as a nurse had also disappeared. However, she must continue to take thyroxine.

There was no miracle, just the clearing of toxic substances from her lymphatic system. Sheila's doctor, although very pleased, quite rightly warned her of the dangers associated with not taking her medication and she was monitored carefully.

Sheila's treatment was several years ago and she still keeps in touch. Blood tests indicate that she still needs her thyroxine but her inhalers have never been reintroduced. Rather than suffering from asthma as was suggested, in this instance, Sheila suffered from congestion of the lymphatics.

Sheila's exercise program progressed very quickly and this is the exception to the rule. Any home treatment should follow the route taken by James, with the suggested frequency of all the exercises, reflexology and massage undertaken in the timescale that is presented. The cleansing program should not be rushed. Please note that

Exercise 7 (lymph drainage of the heart) is to be included at the precise time indicated in the text for James.

HELPFUL HINTS

● Water filters: these filter chlorine from tap water used for drinking and cooking. However, it is beneficial to let water stand to allow the gas to evaporate.

● House plants: these can harbor a fungus on the soil, possibly in the form of white spots. If these spores become air-borne and enter the nasal passage they can cause irritation for the asthmatic. Any areas in the home where condensation is a problem should also be checked for fungus.

● Bicarbonate of soda: One tablespoon of bicarbonate of soda should be added to the final rinse cycle of a washing machine if an excess of chlorine is suspected. Using a non-biological soap powder, 1 egg cup per wash is adequate for normal soiling in most water.

Bicarbonate of soda used around the home can reduce contact with cleaning agents that contain chlorine. Used on a damp cloth or made into a paste, it can clean glass, silver and bathrooms. A handful can be put in the bottom of the dishwasher, and it can also be used to clean the teeth, as some toothpastes contain chlorine.

Many elderly people soak their false teeth in bleach, exposing themselves to chlorine absorption. Some propriety brands of denture cleaner also contain chlorine, therefore cleaning with bicarbonate of soda is preferable. Tea and coffee stains should not be removed from cups and mugs with bleach, as the ceramic material is porous; bicarbonate of soda should be used instead.

● Paper handkerchiefs: one patient eliminated her sinus problems when the fibers from paper handkerchiefs were identified.

● Feather pillows and duvets: most asthmatics are aware that feathers can induce an allergic reaction. Unfortunately, they often go undetected in cases of sinusitis or chronic catarrh.

● Sprays: sprays should be avoided in and around the home. A damp cloth soaked in vinegar can be used to polish furniture and clean windows.

● Oats: porridge made with water or goats milk is beneficial in the morning. It boosts resistance to disease, cleanses the arteries and reduces mucus in the body.

● Liquorice root: this can be beneficial to some people who suffer from breathing problems.

● Ginger root: this is an excellent herb for the respiratory system.

● Oils: add two drops of ginger, one drop of camphor, one drop of eucalyptus and one drop of menthol to 10 ml of base oil and massage into the chest area each night. These oils can also be dropped into a bowl of very hot water and the patient should place a towel over his or her head and inhale the vapor.

Caution: almond oil should be used as the base oil providing the patient doesn't suffer from a nut allergy. All of these suggestions should be checked by using ISR.

● Garlic tablets: these are excellent for respiratory problems but they can contain sulfur and must be checked.

● Some natural foods can trigger an attack of asthma. These include: almond, blackberry, cherry, grapes, peach, pear, strawberry, apricot, apple, rhubarb.

● Sulfite: this is used as a preservative in many foods, including crisps, dried fruits, cooked meat and fish, wines. It can trigger an asthmatic attack, so too can aspirin.

Supplements

● Homeopathy:
  – Bellis perennis: for bronchial plexus
  – Belladonna: mediastinal plexus
  – Micromeria: lungs
  – Spigelia: cardiac ganglion.
● Chamomile tea: soothes, it is antispasmodic and anti-inflammatory.
● Selenium A.C.E.: has been helpful for some asthmatics.

The most common food sensitivities in asthmatics are cows milk and dairy produce, cocoa, onion and tomato.

Magnesium plus vitamin C can be most beneficial for many asthmatics.

Doctor Wright (see p 105) promotes vitamin B12 to restore stomach acid, magnesium supplements for the reduction of muscle spasms (including bronchospasms) plus vitamin B6 to help in the absorption of magnesium.

It might not be beneficial to take all of the supplements mentioned above. The list is to be used as a guide in conjunction with ISR to determine the supplements that are best suited to the individual.

Note: all asthmatics should carry their medication with them at all times regardless of the improvement in their condition. They might be exposed to an irritant without their knowledge and this could trigger an attack.

The reflexology charts and acupuncture points that are relevant for this case study are shown in Figs 12.3 and 12.4 and are to be used in conjunction with ISR in association with the particular lymphatic drainage techniques for integrated therapy.

REFERENCES

The Alternative Health Information Bureau 1995 Nutritional Medicine and Asthma. Alternatives in Health; June/July issue

British Medical Association 1990 Complete family health encyclopaedia. Dorling Kindersley, London

Kokkonen N A 1996 Asthma in children. What Doctors Don't Tell You; 7(4): 8

Millard F P 1922 Applied anatomy of the lymphatics. Australia: International Lymphatic Research Society. (Available from: Health Research, PO Box 850, Pomeroy, Western Australia 99347)

Oschman J 2000 Energy medicine. Harcourt Publishers, London

Randolph T G, Moss R W 1980 Allergies: your hidden enemy. Thorsons, Northampton

Thomas P 2001 Drug additives the not-so inactive ingredients. What Doctors Don't Tell You; 12(5): 2

What Doctors Don't Tell You 2001 Drug additives, the not-so inactive ingredients. What Doctors Don't Tell You; 12(5): August

Wright J 1996 What Doctors Don't Tell You; 7(4)

FURTHER READING

Hanssen M, Marsden J 1984 E is for additives. Thorsons, Northampton

Information about substances used as preservatives can be found online:

Sodium benzoate: www.jtbaker.com/msds/s2930.html
www.hazard.com/msds/tox/f/q28/q184.html

Sodium dichlorisocyanurate:
www.gzchemweek.com/lfchem/products/
sodium-dichlorisocyanurate.htm

Sodium hypochlorite:
http://www.cdc.gov.niosh/ipcs/ipcs1119.html

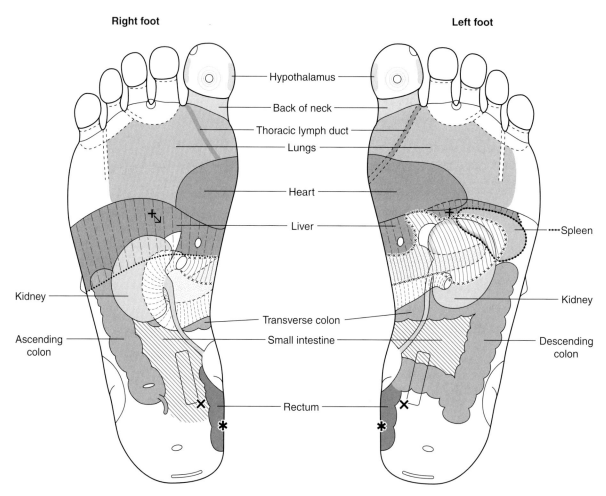

Figure 12.3 Reflexology chart for the liver, kidneys, spleen, heart, lungs, lymph drainage points, lymph cistern, small and large intestines, hypothalamus and pancreas. © F. Fox, used with permission.

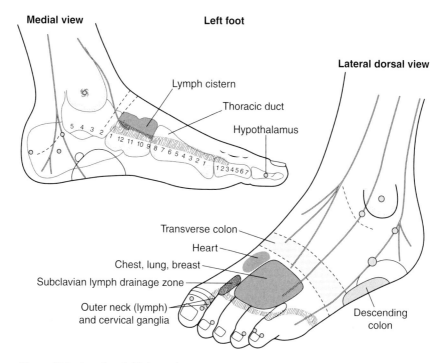

Medial view

Left foot

Lateral dorsal view

Lymph cistern

Thoracic duct

Hypothalamus

Transverse colon

Heart

Chest, lung, breast

Subclavian lymph drainage zone

Outer neck (lymph)
and cervical ganglia

Descending
colon

Figure 12.3 (*continued*). Unless otherwise stated, all reflex zones apply to both feet.

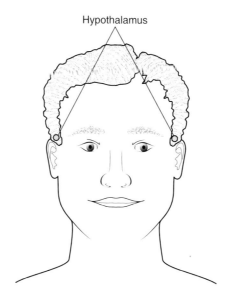

Hypothalamus

Figure 12.4

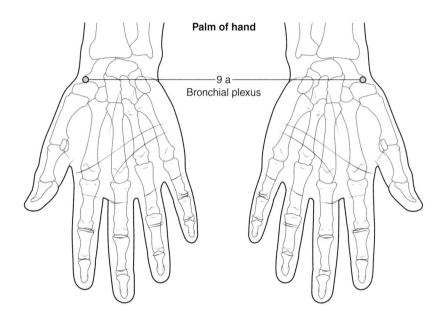

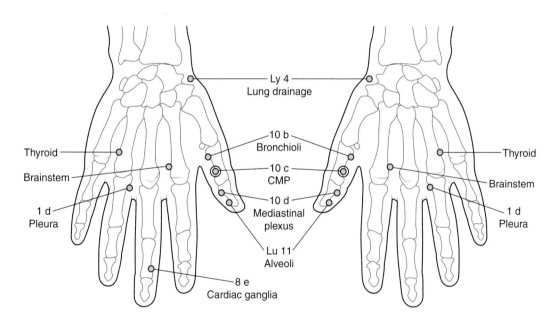

Figure 12.4 (*continued*). Relevant acupuncture points. The points illustrated are for fingertip testing, assessment, and acupressure only. CMP, control measurement point.

13

Metal congestion causing mood swings and reactive hypoglycemia

FIRST VISIT

It has become apparent that the condition hypoglycemia is more widespread than was once thought. For this reason, the following case study is written with patients in mind, in the hope that they will recognize the varying symptoms and feel encouraged to have them analyzed.

Susan was eleven when her concerned mother and father brought her to see me. Her parents were no strangers to me as both had been patients in the past. Susan's mother began to explain why she was concerned about her daughter. Susan apparently lacked concentration and was clumsy, often with outbursts of anger, which were causing problems both at home and in school. She complained of tiredness most mornings and didn't really want to cooperate or take part in any activity. Susan didn't hesitate to let me know that her mother was fussing nor did she attempt to hide her disapproval at sitting in the clinic.

After listening to her mother's account of the situation, which covered this wide range of symptoms and the comparison in concentration to that of her two sisters it was clear why Susan felt that her mother was just complaining. Mother and daughter were definitely not seeing eye-to-eye. As young as she was, Susan wanted to stamp her authority on the situation by explaining she was different to her siblings and liked to do other things! On asking Susan how she was

feeling she just shrugged her shoulders. Her opinion as to why she suffered these symptoms was aimed at her mother as she explained that the constant nagging and complaining was the only problem that she had. After explaining about the treatment, Susan was asked if she wanted to proceed with the tests but her response was just another shrug of the shoulders.

Susan's acupuncture points were duly tested and identified congestion of the ileum. This is the final, longest and narrowest section of the small intestine. It is joined at its upper end to the jejunum and at its lower end to the large intestine. The ileum absorbs nutrients from food that has been digested in the stomach and the first two sections of the small intestine.

Infrequently, the ileum becomes obstructed, for example, by pushing through a weakness in the abdominal wall (hernia) or by becoming caught up with scar tissue following abdominal surgery (British Medical Association 1990, p 564). However, fluoride was the substance identified in Susan's ileum, and was also apparent in her lymphatics, appendix, hypothalamus and abdominal aortic plexus.

Susan's family dentist had apparently recommended fluoride drops, and later tablets, to be given to Susan from a very early age in an attempt to prevent tooth decay. The family also used fluoride toothpaste. Due to the location of the congestion, I enquired if Susan had suffered from pain in her lower back or legs. Suddenly, she became more interested and alert. She explained that during her weekly dancing lesson some leg movements had become difficult to perform and the teacher had become quite cross because they were not difficult to achieve. Identifying the appendix area, Susan was asked if she ever felt any discomfort there. This question again caught her attention. Both mother and daughter explained that she had complained of pain in this region on numerous occasions. The family doctor was unable to identify any abnormality and attributed the pain to the onset of her periods. Congestion in this lower abdominal region usually affects the psoas muscles, causing a spasm, which can throw the body out of alignment and restrict leg movement. Spinal muscles will always be a casualty of this scenario as muscles and ligaments attached to the innominate bones are deprived of correct lymph and venous flow, and they will also spasm. It is conceivable that restrictions imposed by this congestion could be misconstrued in one so young as lack of commitment, particularly if easy exercises couldn't be accomplished.

The abdominal aortic plexus

The abdominal aortic plexus is located in the midabdominal region and is involved in numerous tasks that take place within the body. However, it has become apparent during much investigation using EAV that if this plexus is disturbed by congestion in the adjacent lymphatics, the islets of Langerhans would also be low in energy. For the benefit of the patient,
I will explain the function of these cells.

The islets of Langerhans

The islets of Langerhans are nests of endocrine cells that are embedded in the tissue of the pancreas. They are surrounded by many blood vessels into which they secrete the hormones insulin and glucagon, which regulate the level of glucose in the blood. This task of maintaining normal levels of glucose in the blood is a very

complicated one: The absorption of glucose into body cells (which need the glucose for energy), and into the liver and fat cells for storage, is the responsibility of insulin. If there is a deficiency of insulin, the level of glucose in the blood will become abnormally high, because the body is unable to remove it from the blood and store it. The body's failure to store or use glucose causes weight loss, hunger and fatigue and results in diabetes (British Medical Association 1990, p 348). The normal adult pancreas should contain about 8 mg of insulin and it should be able to produce new insulin to replace what is used every day. The chief factors that make this possible are adequate nerve impulses and blood supply. It would appear that the nerve impulses from the abdominal aortic plexus play a significant part in this process.

On testing Susan's acupuncture points for the islets of Langerhans and pancreas, their energy, although disturbed, was not too low. As a safeguard it was suggested that Susan visit her doctor to have her urine or blood tested to eliminate diabetes mellitus.

Diabetes mellitus, which is too much glucose in the blood, is caused by lack of insulin. The condition is controlled by either self-injections of insulin and/or tablets and diet. Without regular injections of insulin the sufferer lapses into a coma and dies. Hypoglycemia, in a diabetic person, is too little glucose in the blood. This condition causes weakness, confusion, dizziness, sweating and even seizures and unconsciousness. If not treated immediately with either an intake of sugar or an injection of glucose, the sufferer can lapse into a coma, which in extreme cases can lead to death. Disturbances in the careful balance between insulin and glucose can result in either of these two conditions in a diabetic person. It is very important, therefore, that if a patient presents a low energy output for the islets of Langerhans, medical investigations are undertaken as soon as possible.

Another condition that can present when these areas of the body are congested is reactive hypoglycemia or low blood sugar. Unfortunately, this is not identifiable by a simple blood or urine test and is not easily diagnosed.

Reactive hypoglycemia can also give rise to fatigue, weakness, confusion, dizziness and sweating. It is thought that the pancreas releases too much insulin and, as a result, the body and brain are starved of the sugar they need to function correctly. Reactive hypoglycemia can be very debilitating and confusing for the patient so whenever symptoms such as these are presented, and diabetes has been eliminated, this condition must be considered.

The main aim of this treatment session was the identification of toxic matter within the lymphatic system, in the hope that it could be removed from Susan's environment, and to prepare the filters in readiness for the cleansing process. It should not be difficult to remove fluoride, there are, after all, fluoride-free toothpastes on the market, but unfortunately this is not always the case (see Chapter 14). In the meantime, we awaited the results of the blood/urine test for diabetes.

Treatment

For the benefit of patients reading this book who suspect that reactive hypoglycemia might be responsible for their symptoms, the treatment program below can be followed with ease.

Photographs accompany the instructions on how to perform the exercises in Appendix 2.

1. **Reflexology.** To the liver, kidneys, lung, spleen and lymph drainage points (see Fig. 13.3, pp 128–129) and massage above and below the clavicles.
2. **The red light massage.** As the thyroid and parathyroid glands depend upon nerve impulses from the cervical ganglion, it would be most beneficial if this exercise became a daily activity for the prevention of other conditions. For instance, hypothyroidism (which causes tiredness and can contribute to obesity), hyperthyroidism (which can lead to weight loss), osteoarthritis and osteoporosis (which are due to faulty calcium metabolism), can all benefit from this massage. As the heart and lungs also take advantage from the energetic interaction that is encouraged by this massage, it can pay dividends to be rigorous

in its application. It will, however, take about 3 weeks for the nerve impulses from the ganglion to return to normal.

3. **Exercise 1, lymph cistern.**
4. **Do-in.** Gently tap the base of the breast bone and the sides of the rib cage.
5. **Exercise 3, inguinal drain.**
6. **Foot rotation.**
7. **Reflexology.** To the liver, kidneys, lungs, spleen and the lymph drainage points, pancreas, sacroiliac joint, psoas muscles, appendix, adrenal glands and lymph cistern. Massage above and below the clavicles.

This concluded this treatment session until the doctor's report on the urine/blood test for diabetes became available. Reflexology should be completed each evening and the treatment program should be repeated once a week for 2 weeks.

SECOND VISIT

Susan's second visit was much friendlier and she was anxious to talk. All medical tests proved negative, ruling out diabetes. Her parents reported fluctuations in her moods and attitude but she did appear to be walking better. The acupuncture points were still congested, but fluoride was accompanied this visit by the metals chrome, cobalt, nickel and copper. As explained in the previous case studies, when the body detoxifies, it is the surface lymphatics that clear first. The congested deep lymph nodes and vessels might be burdened with different material, so this must be identified and encouraged through the vessels and nodes to be neutralized. As they emerge, these new substances will often stick in the same areas as any previous matter; this might be due to a magnetic imprint or 'photographic negative'. This is particularly true of fluoride in the lymphatics, which appears to be attracted to other materials, making the whole sticky mass difficult to move. Many metals found in the lymphatics are associated with amalgam fillings. However, Susan didn't have any fillings, although she did have a brace on her teeth.

The super snooper (see Chapter 11)

Using the super snooper, the brace in Susan's mouth was identified as a source of the metals identified earlier in parts of her body. EAV and ISR identified the acupuncture points that were being burdened by metals from their low energy readings. When the snooper was placed on the brace, only those acupuncture points where metal had been identified returned to normal. The magnet was making the exact antidote for toxic matter as soon as that substance came within the range of the magnet's field. It appears to work on a similar principle as a homeopathic remedy: producing the mirror image of the magnetic field out of harmony with the magnetic field of the body, thus cancelling out any disharmony. It is now possible to identify any item outside of the body that was responsible for causing distorted energy within. Trials conducted by Fox and me over many years using this method were fascinating, in particular, the tracing of the path metals took once they were inside the body (see Chapter 11). When Susan's parents saw the results of the tests they decided to take her to see the dentist. The permanent brace was removed and replaced by a partial one that was to be worn during the night.

THIRD VISIT

On Susan's third visit, I tested the new brace using the snooper but unfortunately this too contained metal and would have a similar effect on her body. It was quite amazing to discover how her body responded to the metal, and this fact could be demonstrated by using ISR. First, the spasm that was in the webbing of her hand was cleared, leaving the muscle flaccid, which both parents could feel. When the new brace was placed in her other hand the spasm immediately returned and was strong enough to cause Susan discomfort. Both parents were able to feel this change for themselves, which was quite unsettling for them, having informed their dentist that Susan couldn't tolerate metals in her mouth. Admittedly, the amount of metal seemed insignificant but nevertheless it still caused a stress to the immune system and distortion of energy; the brace needed to be removed.

This discovery was unsettling for Susan's parents, and in particular her mother. However, after much deliberation she decided that Susan should continue with the treatments in the hope that any absorption of metal could be kept to a minimum by the treatments, particularly if they were vigilant with the exercises at home. However, the abdominal aortic plexus continued to display a low energy output at each visit, which caused concern. As investigations had ruled out diabetes, the possibility of reactive hypoglycemia (low blood sugar) was considered. Food sensitivity plays a tremendous role in this condition, however, without correct stimulus from the abdominal aortic plexus, this complaint will never be managed.

The offending foods had to be withdrawn from Susan's diet to reduce the stress this imposed upon the pancreas if the energy from the plexus was to be corrected. Susan was tested using ISR. The foods that were identified as being out of harmony with her own energy fields were milk, wheat, coffee, tea, sugar, rice, eggs and carrots. A very restrictive diet for one so young, although coffee, tea, eggs and rice should not pose too much of a problem.

As all foods convert to some form of sugar in the blood, the task of maintaining normal levels is a very complicated one. If the dietary source of sugar is insufficient to maintain normal levels of glucose, the blood should then begin absorbing adequate amounts from its store in the liver where it is known as glycogen. Before glycogen can be utilized, it has to be changed back into glucose. This is activated by the hormone glucagon, which is produced and secreted by the islets of Langerhans in the pancreas, and by other cells scattered throughout the gastrointestinal tract. Its function is to raise the level of sugar in the blood. However, its production is dependent upon the correct stimuli to the gastrointestinal tract as well as from the abdominal aortic plexus. Whenever glucagon is in short supply, the level of glucose in the blood will drop below normal, causing low blood sugar. This can happen if a meal is missed, and is often accompanied by headache.

This situation will usually resolve itself in a healthy person, especially when food is eaten. Unfortunately, reactive hypoglycemia doesn't always respond to food, in fact, some foods make the condition worse and so need to be identified, particularly when disturbances to the abdominal aortic plexus have been identified.

Disturbance to or from the abdominal aortic plexus always involves the carbohydrate function of the pancreas, interfering with the production of enzymes. These enzymes, which are secreted into the gut, are required for digestion of carbohydrates and often proteins. If they are absent then sensitivity or an allergy to foods and other substances can result, which usually has a significant effect on the way the body handles its sugar.

If the nerve supply to the pancreas is overstimulated then too much insulin can be produced. This could be caused by the congested lymphatics in close proximity to a plexus distorting the signals, or be as a direct result from overeating the wrong foods, in particular sugary foods, or a combination of both these factors. The body has a propensity to overcorrect deficiency and if one takes in too much sugar the body will respond by producing insulin to remove the extra sugar from the blood (Mason 1981, p 1). If this happens too often it can cause the pancreas to become 'trigger-happy'. A healthy person with an adequately functioning lymphatic system and whose energy fields are not being distorted can usually adjust to this up-and-down situation. However, others are not so fortunate and the symptoms displayed by Susan will be the result.

It is difficult to decide which malfunction appears first: an allergy or a distorted energy field. Either one might actually be a part of our inheritance and the primary defect. If this is so then the testing of newborn babies for any malfunction or allergy could be of enormous benefit to their future health.

The part diet plays

It has been recognized for some time now that refined carbohydrates are one of the most common contributing factors in reactive hypoglycemia and should be avoided. These are found in white flour, white rice, most convenience foods, snacks and chocolate. Foods containing sugar and glucose are absorbed very quickly in the gut, rapidly increasing blood sugar levels and resulting in excessive production of insulin; the outcome is low blood sugar. When this happens, the body's fuel supply is greatly depleted. Nerve cells and organs struggle to carry out vital functions, especially the job of manufacturing the proteins and other materials needed in the production of muscle and nerve tissues and the enzymes that regulate body functions (Mason 1981, p 1).

Stress

Whenever people are placed under stress, their bodies will give priority to the production of epinephrine (adrenaline). Regardless of whether the stress is caused by fear, hate, anger or worry about tomorrow's bills, the demand on the adrenal glands is the same. The body cannot differentiate between any of these emotions and any sudden emergency. Neither can it proportion the epinephrine output to allow for some figment of the imagination or confrontation with a lion. Because of this, higher amounts of the essential raw materials are needed. When their energy begins to drop, people in this situation will feel worried, or even hatred, for no apparent reason. These emotions, though, will increase their blood sugar levels, which has the effect of pulling sugar directly from the liver and muscles. The blood sugar is increased just as if one ate a candy bar, only the body is supplying the sugar. There are those who suffer from low blood sugar who are actually addicted to worry or hate just as others are addicted to drugs, alcohol or smoking. Anything that causes an increase in blood glucose will at the same time cause a reaction of insulin. The body does not have any way of knowing if the glucose came from sugar, fruit or any other source. Reactive hypoglycemia is a reaction to an increase in blood sugar caused by any stimulant, be it coffee, cigarettes, emotions or pep pills (Mason 1981, pp 32–33).

Undiagnosed hypoglycemia can go on for years, possibly indefinitely, putting tremendous strain on the pancreas without anybody being aware that the symptoms presented here are warning signs. If they are misinterpreted, resulting in misdiagnosis, then the patient will not only be deprived of the appropriate treatment but might receive unnecessary drugs. By not identifying the true cause, the pancreas will continue to be under pressure, and could react by stopping production of insulin altogether. The consequence is diabetes. It is recognized that a diet rich in complex carbohydrates (unrefined foods such as wholemeal flour, brown rice, baked potatoes and pulses), which break down into sugar at a much slower rate than refined carbohydrates, thus reducing the need for the body to produce an excess of insulin. This type of diet would therefore appear to be helpful for anybody suffering from reactive hypoglycemia. However, sensitivities to certain foods, irrespective of carbohydrate content, can have a similar effect to sugar. Elimination of sensitive foods from the diet is the only sensible solution, together with eating small amounts of food every 2 hours. This should prevent massive fluctuations in the level of insulin and glucose and will eventually result in a better state of mind and body. Practising the techniques outlined in the treatment section, particularly Exercises 8 (nerve supply to the islets of Langerhans) and 9 (deep inguinal nodes) will ensure that the lymphatic system, and in particular the abdominal area that contains these vital nerve plexuses, functions to its optimum efficiency. When the energy to the pancreas is restored sufficiently then many of the original food sensitivities will disappear.

Mental function

As the cells of the brain require glucose to function normally, it is hardly surprising that many of the symptoms of hypoglycemia can also be related to mental function. It would therefore be prudent to eliminate reactive hypoglycemia from the many individuals suffering from any form of depression or anxiety before any medication is suggested. Until recently, the only available method of helping to balance the chemistry of the brain was through a variety of drugs, which are inclined to dampen emotional and mental activity but which have undesirable side-effects. Only when scientists started to examine what the brain and nervous system was actually made of did the importance of nutrition become apparent in mental health. For its development, the brain uses more than 60% of all nutrients passed from the mother to the fetus during pregnancy. Even in a mature adult, about 30% of all energy derived from food is used by the brain.

Modern-day living exposes people to many chemicals that interfere with how the nutrients from food work. These 'antinutrients' include certain kinds of food additives, household chemicals, drugs and inhaled pollutants from smoking, exhaust fumes and industrial pollution.

Carl Pfeiffer, an American doctor and biochemist at the Brain BioCenter in New Jersey, classified glucose intolerance as one of the five main underlying factors in schizophrenia. Psychiatric symptoms of glucose intolerance have been noted to include unsociable or antisocial behavior, phobias, suicide attempts, nervous breakdown and psychosis, hyperactivity, depression, eating disorders, fatigue, learning disabilities and premenstrual tension. Specific diets and nutrients resulted in improvement in certain types of mental illness. Many of these symptoms are exhibited as a result of a lack of a continuous supply of glucose to the brain, which is necessary for the mind and body to work properly.

Treatment

Appendix 2 contains photographs and instructions to the patient on how to perform the exercises in the following list.

1. **Reflexology.** To the liver, kidneys, spleen, lungs and massage above and below the clavicles.
2. **Exercise 1, lymph cistern.**
3. **Do-in.** To the bottom of the sternum then up the center of the sternum and to the base of the rib cage on both sides.

4. **Self-help abdominal massage.**
5. **Foot rotation.**
6. **Exercise 8, to stimulate the nerve supply to the islets of Langerhans and the carbohydrate function of the pancreas.**
7. **Exercise 9, deep inguinal nodes.** Exercises 8 and 9 can be of benefit where frequent urination is a problem as they can improve the performance of the organs in the lower abdomen.
8. **Do-in.** To the base of the sternum.
9. **Exercise 4, the four-step exercise.**
10. **Do-in.** To the base of the sternum.
11. **Reflexology.** To the liver, kidneys, spleen, lungs, pancreas, adrenal glands, appendix, gall bladder and lymph cistern (see Fig. 13.3, p 128).

Gall bladder exercise

Insulin-dependent diabetics should not use this technique.

This exercise can help enormously when reactive hypoglycemia is suspected.

Lean forward and, with the fingertips of one or both hands, press up under the rib cage below the right breast to compress the gall bladder (Fig. 13.1). Then push out the abdomen against the fingertips once or twice.

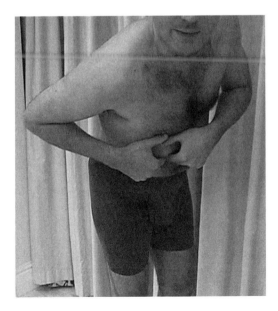

Figure 13.1 Gall bladder exercise.

Adrenal glands

As cortisone and epinephrine can raise the level of sugar in the blood and are produced by the adrenal glands, they are always included in the reflexology chart for reactive hypoglycemia, but Exercises 8 and 9 also help to regulate the functions that are performed by these glands (see Chapter 16 for adrenal function test).

FOURTH VISIT

On testing Susan's acupuncture points, metals were yet again causing congestion and, unfortunately, there was additional friction between mother and daughter. When looking in on Susan before going to bed, her parents had found that the tooth brace was lying on the pillow. On some occasions Susan was awakened to replace the brace and the old tensions returned, with mother accusing daughter of removing the brace on purpose before she went to sleep and Susan categorically denying the fact.

As the brace contained a substance that Susan's body didn't want, it was natural that it should try to expel it, which it was able to do during the night. It was fascinating that Susan's body would not tolerate the metal in the brace, however small the amount, and absorption during the night from this brace was as detrimental to her body as it was from the previous brace. If her body was to be free from the distortion caused by these harmful metals, then that exposure must be removed. As the brace was primarily for cosmetic reasons, Susan and her parents decided to dispense with it completely. By removing the offending substance, distortion of vital energy would be reduced and, hopefully, she could start on the road to recovery. It is worth mentioning at this point that the body must never be underestimated in its ability to find a solution to heal itself, which it does by removing an irritant in any way it can. The brace on the pillow was no coincidence; it is as significant as a bout of diarrhea in the removal of harmful bacteria. By removing an irritant the body will require little assistance in the healing process.

FIFTH VISIT

Six weeks later mother and daughter walked into the clinic and reported a significant change. Susan's energy level in particular was commented upon, and the problem with her lower spine was non-existent. Her moods were better but she still suffered from the occasional headache. The acupuncture readings mirrored this improvement. There was no reason to suspect that this improvement should not continue.

During the many treatment sessions that followed over the years, Susan's symptoms fluctuated with the removal of many substances. The metal that lingered in Susan's case was cobalt. Other substances included the childhood vaccines for tuberculosis, the BCG. Each substance, as it came to the surface, brought a deterioration in behavior and lack of concentration. This was accompanied by familiar joint and back pain, which Susan could identify and rectify at home using the many exercises and reflexology charts. As cobalt is a left-drift metal, it will exit the body on the left side. It was very important, therefore, that Susan concentrated very carefully on her left kidney and left lobe of her liver to ensure its speedy and safe removal from her body.

After each visit, which Susan likened to having a vacuum cleaner go through her whole system, she said that she felt wonderful. By the age of eighteen, Susan was free from all the harmful metals and fluoride. It was very obvious that she was in control of herself and enjoying life. When Susan's mother telephoned to make an appointment for Susan before her final exams, she told of her great pleasure in the transformation in her daughter's attitude. Personality changes were reported with sustained periods of concentration. There appeared to be a steady flow of energy rather than the highs and lows that were common at the beginning. I too saw the change and was thrilled with Susan's obvious pleasure when she entered the clinic for her treatment. She was looking forward to finishing her studying although, like most students, she was very nervous and apprehensive about the exams.

Susan's sensitivities had diminished over the years and she was learning to identify the changes to her moods after she ate something that was not suitable for her. Most hypoglycemics will actually crave the food that causes their low blood sugar, similar to an alcohol or drug addict. Unfortunately, reactive hypoglycemia does not receive the same level of support, although it can also be debilitating and very disruptive to many people.

Three months after her last treatment, a very excited Susan telephoned the clinic. Not only had she passed her exams but she had come top in one subject. Some weeks later, Susan's parents visited and were delighted to tell how one of Susan's tutors had spoken to them about her improvement, in particular her concentration and application, and how, some years previously, he would never have thought her capable of receiving such high marks!

Susan is now working, enjoying herself to the full and still practising reflexology and the breathing techniques to help keep it that way.

SELF-HELP

Eating small amounts of food every 2 hours helps to make glucose more readily available from the gut throughout the day. Follow Susan's treatment program twice a week for 6 weeks, with massage to the relevant reflexology points for 15 minutes each day. After these 6 weeks try and establish your own routine. This program of exercises will enable you to maintain a balance in blood sugar levels providing all of the offending substances have been removed from your diet and environment.

Certain amino acids have a specific action upon the metabolism of glucose. L-glutamic acid, L-lysine, glycine and L-tyrosine, taken with vitamins B1, B2, B6 and C, are reported by many nutritionists to effectively relieve symptoms of low blood sugar. You might want to try these supplements.

The rutin found in buckwheat is also good for low blood sugar, and sensitivity to buckwheat is uncommon.

When blood sugar drops, blood pressure often rises. For raised blood pressure, practise this

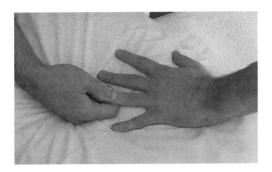

Figure 13.2   Acupressure to reduce hypertension.

massage to the ring finger of the left hand: Enclose this finger between the thumb and index finger of your right hand. From the second joint, massage downwards to the nail (Fig. 13.2). Also, practise the following exercise:

Exercise 6, the brainstem.

Take miso each morning and evening and drink eight glasses of water a day for 3 days after lymphatic drainage, to help the body eliminate the toxins.

The Bach Flower Remedies: Rescue remedy, Centaury or Chestnut Bud can be helpful. They should be tested using ISR.

Magnesium phosphate helps to calm the system. If food testing is not a possibility, it would be advisable to avoid all stimulants, including tea, coffee and nicotine, and to limit alcohol consumption. Paying particular attention to the food chart in Chapter 14, p 138, it might be advisable to remove potatoes and carrots from the diet. But do try to master ISR.

Although diet is crucial in the management of many debilitating illnesses, I cannot stress too strongly the importance of balance. There is no doubt that adhering to a restricted diet can

enable organs of the body to heal, thereby encouraging normal function. A diet with minor adjustments can be managed more easily than a severely restricted one, especially over long periods. Therefore the diet must be monitored rigorously, by rechecking the sensitivities regularly, especially in the young and elderly. Very restricted diets can be harmful, and often lead to more sensitivity, especially if the body is not being supplied with vital nutrients. In some instances, food sensitivities can cause major health problems, leaving no choice but to avoid the offending food indefinitely. Children, in most cases, bounce back to health quickly and their bodies recover rapidly. Adults, however, recover at a slower pace, depending on the amount of damage caused by the offending substances, be they chemical, metal, food or malfunctioning energy fields. Therefore sensitivities can persist.

The reflexology charts and acupuncture points that are relevant for this case study are shown in Figs 13.3 and 13.4 and are to be used in conjunction with ISR and lymphatic drainage techniques.

REFERENCES

British Medical Association 1990 Complete family health encyclopaedia. Dorling Kindersley, London
Mason C F 1981 The methyl approach to hypoglycemia. Mato Laboratory, Vancouver, Canada

FURTHER READING

Budd M 1983 Low blood sugar. Thorsons, Northampton
Erdmann R 1988 Overcoming memory problems. Enzyme Process (UK), Spalding, Lincolnshire
Morter M T 1991 Correlative urinalysis. Thorsons, Northampton

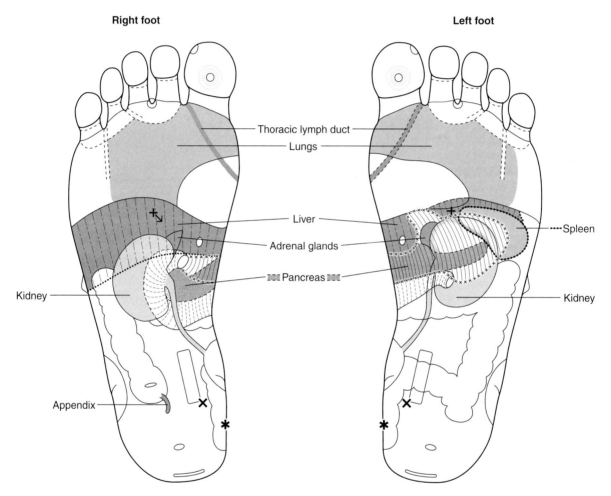

Figure 13.3 Reflexology chart for the liver, kidneys, spleen, lungs, lymph drainage points, pancreas, adrenal glands, appendix, gall bladder and lymph cistern. © F. Fox, used with permission.

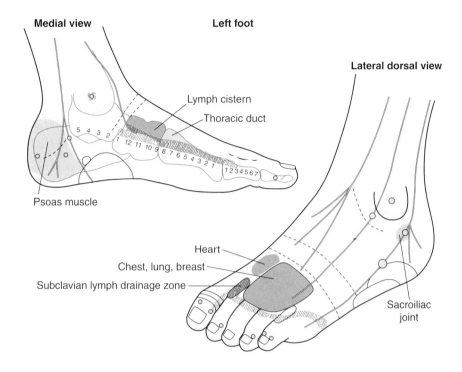

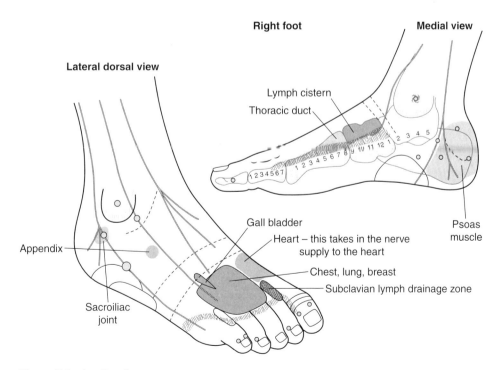

Figure 13.3   (*continued*).

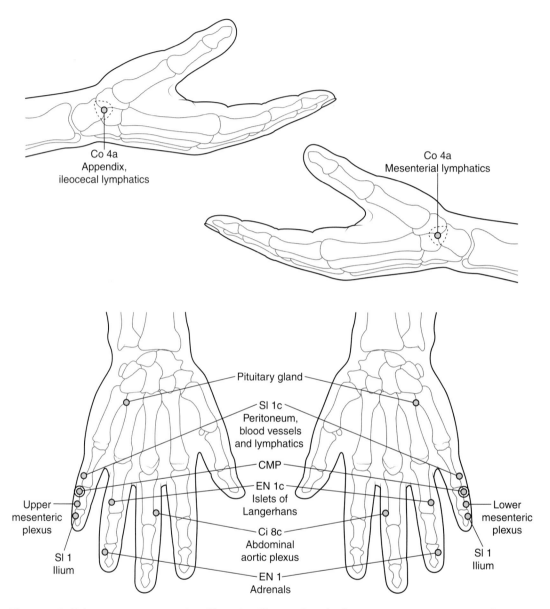

Figure 13.4 Relevant acupuncture points. The points illustrated are for fingertip testing, assessment, and acupressure only. CMP, control measurement point.

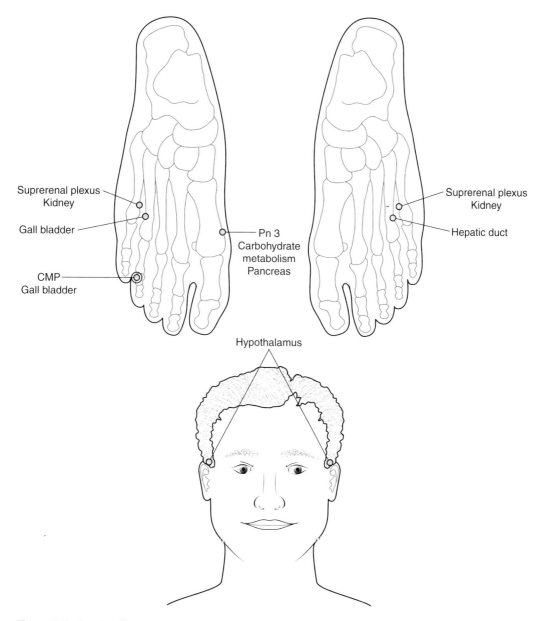

Figure 13.4 (*continued*).

14

Diabetes

FIRST VISIT

In 1990, Monica, a mother of two, rang distraught, to say that Sally, her daughter of ten, had been diagnosed as diabetic and was in hospital. Sally's hospital doctor had given permission for me to see her, if I was agreeable. Monica had been a patient of mine many years previously, and had found integrated therapy to be very successful for a back condition. Other members of her family had enjoyed equal success with a variety of symptoms, so she was hopeful I might be able to help Sally.

Upon testing the acupuncture points of Sally's lymphatic system I found fluoride distorting the electrical output of the pancreas, the small and large intestine, pituitary gland, hypothalamus and abdominal aortic plexus.

Sally was born when the family was living in an area where fluoride had been added to the water. However, not only is fluoride in some water supplies, but it is also found in toothpaste, some soaps and soap powders, insecticides, some antiseptics, relaxants and refrigerants. It used to be used as a constituent of propellants, but these are now reported to be fluoride free. The areas of congestion identified in Sally's body often give rise to other symptoms too: aching muscles, flu-like symptoms and joint pains, possibly including back pain. If any patient presents with this set of symptoms it would be prudent to investigate pancreatic energy levels.

Diabetes mellitus

Diabetes can be brought on by damage to the pituitary gland or, more commonly, by a malfunction of the pancreas. Symptoms include frequent urination and continual thirst. Also, because the tissues are starved of glucose, the person can feel tired and apathetic, and might lose a lot of weight as the body breaks down fat and muscle for energy. Other likely symptoms are lowered resistance to infection (especially urinary tract infections) cramp, tingling in the hands and feet, and blurred vision. In young people diabetes can onset in a matter of months. Once diagnosed, hospitalization is essential to assess and monitor the level of insulin required. Because the pancreas secretes insufficient insulin (or none at all) in diabetes, the cells cannot absorb energy-giving glucose from the blood, nor can the liver absorb and store it. Therefore excess glucose is excreted in urine, which has to have a higher water content than normal to carry it. So urination is frequent and passed in large amounts.

Fluoride

Scientists and medical experts argue that fluoridation of public water supplies helps to reduce tooth decay. Apparently, areas where this has already been done confirm this. It would appear, therefore, that to introduce fluoridation of water to other areas is the only rational thing to do and for 30 years successive British governments have promoted the fluoridation of water as a means of combating dental decay. When Norman Fowler was Health and Social Services Secretary, he announced the government's intention to introduce legislation, commissioning the power of water authorities to add fluoride to the water supply, when the parliamentary timetable permitted.

Natural fluoride

It was in Texas (in the 1940s) where the connection between fluoride and teeth was first noted. The area reported naturally high levels of fluoride in its water supply, and a population that required little or no dental treatment. This prompted government officials to investigate the possibility of using the excess fluoride that was available as a waste product from the fertilizer industry. Unfortunately, the product that the water authorities then added to the water supply was not the same as that originally found in Texas. The natural constituent of the water in Texas was calcium fluoride, which leached out of rock formations in the Texas area (Fox, unpublished work).

Fluorine

Fluorine is the most electronegative element and the strongest oxidizing agent. It exists as a pungent yellow gas or as a liquid. It is used to produce fluoride and, in its anionic form, it is found in fluoridation compounds for drinking water and in toothpaste.

Although minimal amounts of fluorine serve as essential nutrition, excessive amounts are highly toxic. This is true of all elements that lack an electron on the outer ring and therefore latch on to other elements, especially hydrogen: this makes them very 'sticky'. Fluorine, chlorine, bromine and iodine are such substances; they are known as hydrogen halides. Because of their great chemical activity, all hydrogen halides are very poisonous, with fluorine being the most deadly of them all; in fact, it is the most powerful

oxidizing substance in the chemical world. Fluorine dissolved in water forms hydrofluoric acid, which is extremely dangerous.

Many insecticides contain compounds of fluorine and are considered safe for consumption, provided a given time has elapsed since their application. Fruit and vegetables are apparently sprayed for public protection but if hydrofluoric acid forms in water from fluorine this could be dangerous. Fluorine compounds in toothpaste and mouthwashes break down plaque (through oxidation) by destroying the natural habitat for bacteria. Fluorine also attacks and oxidizes many metals, and also glass.

Neurotoxicity of fluoride

In the journal *Fluoride,* in 1996, Dr Phyllis Mullenix recorded her unease over the lack of investigation into the possible link between fluoride and effects on the central nervous system (CNS), including the feasibility that fluoride exposure is linked with subtle brain dysfunction. She draws attention to reports from Chinese investigators that high levels of fluoride in drinking water (3–11 parts per million) affect the CNS without deviation or sign of causing the physical deformities of skeletal fluorosis. A further research report from China in November 1995 indicates adverse neurological effects on the brain from fluoride exposure. This work suggests that children with dental fluorosis are at greater risk of decreased mental acuity. The adverse effects of fluorides occur after ingestion, as it can reach every cell of the body, and can especially damage the bones and teeth. It has been linked to hip fractures and half of all ingested fluoride remains in the skeletal system and accumulates with age (Fluoride Action Network 2000).

In London, researchers at King's College have also conducted much research and have shown that fluoride forms very strong hydrogen bonds with amides, which are formed when amino acids join together to form a protein. If the protein is distorted, the body's immune system no longer recognizes it, treats it as a foreign protein and will try to destroy it, which in turn triggers allergic skin or gastrointestinal reactions (Jones 1999). Pharmaceutical drugs including steroids, antibiotics and even some anesthetics, contain fluoride (Gotzche 1992). In fact, the chemical name for Prozac is fluoxetine hydrochloride. This drug was licensed in 1987 and it is estimated to have been used to treat half a million people in the UK alone.

An agricultural catalogue in 1995 listed 2700 products containing organic fluoride for farm use. The impact of fluoride on crops, soil, animals and workers and those who eat this produce must be quite significant, but as yet there doesn't appear to be any facility for the monitoring of its safety level of toxicity in the individual. This is indeed required if, after it enters the body and makes its way into the gastrointestinal tract, fluoride can be absorbed, along with other proteins, into the bloodstream via the portal vein and liver. Alternatively, it could stick somewhere as a reject protein and damage the immune system with its rogue magnetic field.

Energy fields in crisis

The book *Energy medicine* (Oschman 2000, p 69) mentions the work of Yoshio Manaka, who states that there are many unknown communication circuits and informational units within the body. Basically, when you touch the human body you connect with an intricate network of continuously interconnected components (Oschman 2000, p 20).

Burr, in his investigations into the detection of cancer (Burr 1957), was convinced that diseases would show up in the energy field before symptoms of pathology, such as tumors. His theory was that if the disturbed energy fields could be detected and then restored to normal, then pathology could be prevented. Although his work at the time was met with much scepticism, particularly the existence of acupuncture meridians and points, Voll, and later Schimmel, confirmed his findings (Oschman 2000). Bergsmann & Wooley-Hart (1973) demonstrated the increased conductance of inflammatory conditions of patients using liver 8, located on the knee. They confirmed that this point on the knee

was 18 times higher in patients with diagnosed cirrhosis of the liver than in patients with no liver disease.

This validation that any liver dysfunction, or for that matter any dysfunction, within the body can be viewed and assessed at various lookout points on the body well away from the actual physical structure is reliable and repeatable. The electrical energy that is produced by all living matter is no different from any other kind of electricity and the body's circuit can certainly be measured. The facility to measure the vibrations of every function within the human body can indeed change the face of diagnosis with its non-invasive approach and its offer of prevention. Identifying the dysfunction and the cause is fascinating, as the living matrix is a continuous, vibrant, interconnecting web and is dependent upon the integrated activities of all of the components.

Fluorine, being a powerful chemical activist, has the potential to disrupt the fine balance of this intricate network. Consequently, pathology will be prevented only when this balance has been restored by the removal of this harmful substance from the tissues and cells.

The late Dr G.L. Waldbott, a well-known authority on fluorides, said, 'It is difficult for doctors not to confuse some diseases – arthritis in particular – with fluoride poisoning, their symptoms being so alike' (Waldbott 1979).

John Yiamouyiannis, a biochemist from Chicago, described as the world's leading authority on the biological effects of fluoride, states that:

Fluoride damages the body's repair and rejuvenation capacities, there is no safe level … Stomach and bowel disorders are the main characteristics of fluoride intolerance. Even small amounts of fluoride can form hydrofluoric acid in the stomach producing gastric pains, nausea and vomiting, putting young children in particular at risk. Fluoride tablets can cause gastric haemorrhages; in one instance, a 9-year-old boy sustained such damage that large parts of his stomach had to be removed.
(Yiamouyiannis 1999)

Many parents actively encourage very young children to suck on a toothbrush laden with flavored toothpaste in the hope of developing good dental hygiene. To avoid permanent tooth discoloration, the Canadian Dental Association advises against fluoride supplement use for children before their permanent teeth have grown. Studies show that tooth decay is declining in both fluoridated and non-fluoridated areas while dental fluoroisi (white spotted, yellow or brown stained and sometimes crumbly teeth) is increasing, more so in fluoridated areas (Fluoride Action Network 2000). Although dental hygiene should be encouraged from an early age, an overload of fluoride in toothpaste is not the answer if a child is likely to swallow it, particularly if that child is sensitive to the substance. A legacy of fluoride can be dangerous, so for this reason identification of sensitivity to the substance is more important than establishing early dental hygiene.

Sally's first treatment

Sally's blood was being monitored regularly by the hospital staff, along with her food. After identifying fluoride as being present in the lymphatics, the next task was to try and eliminate it. Before starting massage it was explained to Monica that any treatment could alter the balance of Sally's sugar levels and, for this reason, it was very important that the medical team be alerted to this possibility.

Full details of how to perform the following exercises can be found in Appendix 1.

1. **Reflexology.** To the liver, kidneys, spleen, lungs, lymph drainage points and pancreas, followed by massage above and below the clavicles (see Fig. 14.1, pp 142–143).
2. **Exercise 1, lymph cistern.**
3. **Abdominal massage.**
4. **Exercise 1, lymph cistern.**
5. **Do-in.** To the bottom of the sternum and below the clavicles either side of the sternum.
6. **Reflexology.** As above.

It was explained to Monica that she must continue the treatment by massaging the reflex zones on Sally's feet twice a day. I stayed at the hospital until Monica felt confident with the procedure and Sally compared the pressure of her mother's thumbs to mine.

I received a telephone call from Monica the next day. Within an hour of my leaving the hospital, Sally didn't feel well. Upon checking her blood levels the staff discovered her blood sugar had dropped considerably, which caused quite a panic. The insulin needed to stabilize Sally was considerably less than had been required prior to the treatment. This reduced level of insulin remained constant until I paid another visit to the hospital, when similar results warranted a further reduction in insulin. Once again, the new level of insulin was established and the medical team involved with Sally was delighted with her stability: she required minimal medical intervention. Sally was discharged from hospital and the parents were given a tremendous amount of support, which included regular hospital appointments and visits to the home by medical personnel. A support group telephone number with much advice on activities and the like was also available, and the family soon realized that having a diabetic child was relatively common, so they felt less isolated. I visited the family at home, where they were continuing to use reflexology, and instructed Monica on the techniques of abdominal massage. Sally was also tested for food sensitivity and found to be intolerant of potatoes, white flour, sugar, monosodium glutamate, tea, coffee, carrots and preservatives; she was particularly sensitive to benzoate. Monica removed all of these substances from Sally's diet immediately.

Not long after the change in diet, Monica contacted Sally's medical team to tell them that Sally was coping without insulin. It was now more important then ever to monitor blood sugar levels. I was impressed with the dedication of this family towards the treatments and massage. Under the circumstances, however, it was understandable that the medical profession was cautious of this approach to insulin management in one so young. Although Sally's parents were very confident and capable, this news unsettled them, as they sought and wanted approval from the medical profession for this integrated route that they were taking. Sally and her parents accepted the fact that she was diabetic with or without the need for insulin. For this reason, her blood was monitored like any other diabetic person. Small amounts of insulin had to be administered on a few occasions but, health- and weight-wise, Sally couldn't have been better. On more than one occasion, the doctor who saw Sally at the diabetic clinic commented on her good health, steady weight and manageability of the condition, expressing admiration, although quizzical at times over the insulin levels. However, some months later, I had a telephone call one Sunday morning from Monica, asking if I could see Sally, whose blood sugar level had suddenly shot up, requiring insulin to be reintroduced. Upon testing Sally, chlorine was found in almost all of the acupuncture points that had exhibited low energy when she first visited me.

Sally had been swimming with the school on Friday, and also with friends on Saturday. The chlorine appeared to be affecting her pancreas in the same way as fluoride. Her body obviously wasn't able to handle the amount of chlorine that she had absorbed through her skin from the water. When insulin had been reintroduced and the frequency of reflexology and massage increased, it was not long before the familiar pattern repeated itself and – eventually – Sally was able to manage without her insulin again. Family discussions were conducted regarding this new discovery and the limitations this imposed on one so young if the swimming baths were banned. Perhaps swimming with the school should be abandoned but occasional trips to the swimming baths with friends allowed as an alternative. This would permit more time for showering the chlorinated water from the hair and body – a luxury not afforded during a school visit. There are alternatives to chlorine for the use in swimming pools but these substitutes are rather more expensive. Without investigation it is impossible to know if they would affect Sally in a similar way as chlorine. (You might remember that chlorine was indicated as a hormone disrupter in Chapter 9.)

The teenage years approached and Sally became reluctant to conform to any rules or regulations. She was no longer handling the restrictions of being a diabetic and she did not want other limitations, including a ban on swimming. Family commitments meant that Monica couldn't always buy organic food and Sally, who had missed her crisps, chips and potatoes, began to slacken her diet. As the restricted diet became less restricted, insulin became a daily event, although – according to her medical team – Sally's dosage was still on the low side.

I saw Sally again a year or two later, when the sugar levels were inconsistent yet again and the level of insulin needed was on the high side. This time it was cobalt that was affecting the pituitary gland and pancreas. This was coming from a tooth brace (see Chapter 13). Being a little older at this stage, Sally realized the importance of a stable blood sugar level and was more diligent in complying with her treatment. Luckily, the brace was needed for only a short time and Sally's blood sugar levels stabilized again when this metal was removed from her mouth.

CLAIRE'S STORY

Claire was eighteen and about to go off to university when she was diagnosed as being diabetic. Similarities between her case and that of Sally were very obvious: not only was fluoride the main component but the food sensitivities too were remarkably similar. Potatoes caused noticeable alterations in blood sugar levels in both cases. Once Claire accepted and came to terms with her diabetes the condition was handled extremely well. She thrived on her restricted diet, which gave extra energy and wellbeing, challenging any restraints the condition imposed. She too was able to reduce her insulin. It was also quite fascinating to listen to this young woman tell how she had never felt so well with an abundance of energy to rival the healthiest person.

THE SIMILARITIES BETWEEN DIABETES AND REACTIVE HYPOGLYCEMIA

The similarities in food sensitivity in people with diabetes and people with reactive hypoglycemia led to further investigation. This was of particular interest to me because my son Gary had a sensitivity to potatoes, which do appear to be a common denominator in both conditions. When Gary was very young he suffered chronic migraine attacks for no apparent reason. Medical investigations drew a blank. After much exploration it was discovered that he was suffering from reactive hypoglycemia and an array of food sensitivities, which included potato. From a diabetic standpoint, Sally's insulin was not needed on a daily basis until she reintroduced potato into her diet.

If Gary eats potatoes (or carrots) it results in him having very little energy and wanting to fall asleep; a migraine often follows. However, omitting carrot and potato from his diet at an early age, combined with lymphatic drainage was instrumental in the demise of his migraine attacks.

Food sensitivity plays a far bigger role in the management of both diabetes and reactive hypoglycemia than is realized and people with undiagnosed, and therefore untreated, reactive hypoglycemia could be just one step away from developing diabetes.

This particular physical therapy produces strong biomagnetic fields that induce healing within the body. A leading medical researcher has confirmed that energy fields can initiate a healing process in the body even in patients unhealed for 40 years (Oschman 2000, p 90). Once offending foodstuffs are removed from the diet of the patient and the lymphatic system has been encouraged to function to its optimum level of efficiency, free-flowing energy opens the channels for intercommunication and therefore repair. Used in the management of both diabetes and reactive hypoglycemia this integrated therapy maintains the health of the pancreas. Further trials are needed to establish the correlation if any, between hypoglycemia, diabetes and this particular integrated therapy. In any event, diabetics who are treated using this technique respond favorably and it is not unusual for their medication to be significantly reduced.

Carbohydrates

In a paper published in 1985 and entitled *Carbohydrates: new findings could change the way you eat*, Janet Hobson states that potatoes release carbohydrates into the blood as fast as sweets do. Throughout most of the twentieth century, nutritionists have accepted two important notions about the digestion of sugars and starches: simple sugars such as sucrose and honey break down quickly; complex carbohydrates such as the starch in wheat, corn and potatoes break down slowly. These concepts have supported millions of carefully planned school lunches and hospital trays and influenced countless personal decisions about what to eat before strenuous exercise or a day at work. Simple sugars should be eaten for quick energy and complex carbohydrates for long-lasting energy, has been the code of belief.

Because of the composition of carbohydrates, nutritionists have thought that they break down and enter the bloodstream more slowly than sugars and laboratory tests have even confirmed this hypothesis. So, 'sugars fast, starches slow' has always been the train of thought, as the following article points out. In 1977, Phyllis Crapo, a dietician at Stanford University, carried out some interesting work. It all came about because she was disturbed by something she'd heard during a lecture:

The lecturer said he was sceptical about the sugars–starches dietary dogma. The human gut, he said, contains so many billions of enzyme molecules, targeted to break carbohydrates down, that there is no reason to think this breakdown happens slowly. Instead, the lecturer suggested, the abundant enzymes will attack the group at once, cleaving it into thousands of glucose boxes simultaneously, thereby flooding the gut and, in turn the bloodstream, with the body's favourite fuel. (Hobson 1985)

This disturbed Crapo because of its implications for diabetics. She was worried that the information she and other advisers had been giving out to patients was misleading – namely that it is preferable to eat complex carbohydrates as opposed to simple so as to avoid acute rises in blood glucose levels. As Janet Hopson continues, Crapo, along with two physicians who specialized in treating diabetics, devised an experiment to test this theory. They recruited 16 healthy volunteers and gave each of them a set of five rather unusual breakfasts. On one morning each received lemon-flavored water containing 50 g (about one-quarter of a cup) of pure glucose. Other mornings they ate either plain boiled rice, canned corn, a plain baked potato or white bread, each serving containing an equivalent of 50 g of glucose tied up in starch molecules. The researchers then took blood samples at intervals for 3 hours and tested for the insulin and blood glucose levels. To everyone's surprise, the foods produced a hierarchy of effects. The pure glucose, of course, gave the highest peaks of blood glucose and insulin. But potato starch had effects very similar to pure glucose, while corn and rice showed lower peaks and bread produced some intermediate effects. Clearly, some starches can break down very fast. Subsequent tests were conducted using starchy foods on diabetic patients, who showed blood sugar responses similar to those of the healthy volunteers, but a bit exaggerated. Although the foods were tested alone and not as part of a meal, certain items may be worth considering. The results are shown in Table 14.1.

Although dieticians and doctors were naturally cautious when carrot was removed from Gary's diet, the results speak for themselves.

Gary was always hungry and, quite often to keep him going until dinnertime, I would peel a carrot for him to eat, until I discovered a pattern emerging. He would have a sudden burst of energy, which could last for half an hour then, just as suddenly, become very tired and often fall asleep. When I tried to waken him for dinner he would be so sleepy that he wouldn't want to eat; yet he had been ravenous an hour earlier. However, his sister had no such reaction, but didn't suffer from reactive hypoglycemia.

Table 14.1 Starch content of different foods*

Food	Starch content*
Bread – white	69
Bread – wholewheat	72
Carrots	92
Cornflakes	80
Glucose	100
Maltose	105
Milk – skim	32
Milk – whole	34
Oatmeal	49
Peanuts	13
Potato chips	51
Potatoes – instant	80
Potatoes – new	70
Rice – brown	66
Rice – white	72
Soya beans	15
Spaghetti – white	50
Spaghetti – wholewheat	42

* The higher the number, the faster the food is converted into glucose.

Preservatives were also substances that Gary couldn't tolerate and they had to be removed from his diet and body. When this cleansing process was completed he became free from migraine attacks.

Treatment

Caution:

1. On no account must the following lymphatic drainage exercises be used as a substitute for insulin.

2. It is vital that diabetic patients check with their therapist and doctor before embarking on any of the exercise steps.

3. All diabetic patients must be made aware of the possibility of hyperinsulinism. Monitoring blood glucose levels after following any part of this therapy program is vital. Diabetic patients would be well advised to read Chapter 13, which will equip them with further information regarding many issues contained within this chapter.

1. Reflexology. To the liver, kidneys, spleen, lungs, lymph drainage points, eye points, pancreas, adrenal glands and lymph cistern (see Fig. 14.1, pp 142–143). Followed by massage above and below the clavicles.

2. **Exercise 1, lymph cistern.**
3. **Do-in.** Gently to the sides of the rib cage.
4. **Self-help abdominal massage technique.**
5. **Repeat Exercise 1, lymph cistern.**
6. **Exercise 4, the four-step exercise.** This helps to stimulate the nerve supplies of the celiac plexus, abdominal aortic plexus, solar plexus, duodenum and jejunum and decongests the superior mesenteric lymph nodes in the epigastrium. It is best performed by the patient under the guidance of the therapist, but can be repeated at home.
7. **Exercise 8.** To clear the nerve supply to the islets of Langerhans and the carbohydrate function of the pancreas. The abdominal aortic plexus is proximal to the second joint on the medial side of the third finger. The abdominal pair of plexuses control carbohydrate metabolism via the pancreas and the production of insulin and glucagon by the islets of Langerhans.
8. **Foot rotation.**
9. **Repeat Exercise 1, lymph cistern.**
10. **Exercise 9.** To clear the deep inguinal nodes.
11. **Repeat Exercise 1, lymph cistern.**
12. **Do-in.** To the base of the sternum and the sides of the rib cage.
13. **Repeat Exercise 1, lymph cistern.** Three more times.
14. **Do-in.** To the base of the sternum and both sides of the rib cage.
15. **Reflexology.** To the liver, kidneys, spleen, lungs, lymph drainage points, pancreas, adrenal glands, pituitary gland, eye points, small and large intestines and gall bladder (see Fig. 14.1, pp 142–143). Massage above and below the clavicles then repeat reflexology to the liver, kidneys, spleen and lungs.

These exercises usually clear the abdominal aortic plexus and correct the nerve supply to the pancreas and islets of Langerhans. I would recommend that the patient be given a chart for relexology to be performed each evening until their next appointment. Steps from the above program should be performed once a week for the first month, providing that reflexology is a nightly ritual. This usually allows sufficient time to jump-start the interconnecting energy fields into action. The program can then be reduced, depending upon the requirement of each patient, under the guidance of the therapist.

Patient's guide

- The skin of diabetic patients can be very dry and thin. Care must be taken during massage or reflexology.
- Drink eight glasses of purified water each day for three days after lymphatic drainage exercises to help the liver and kidneys eliminate the toxins.
- If for any reason food sensitivities cannot be established, it would be advisable for the patient to avoid all stimulants, which include tea, coffee and nicotine, and to limit alcohol consumption. Paying particular attention to Table 14.1, it might also be advisable to remove potatoes and carrots from the diet.
- **Chromium:** is a trace element. Dr Stephen Davies (1987) has reported that it allows insulin to work properly. Brewer's yeast is a good source of chromium, providing a sensitivity to yeast is not a problem; black pepper and wheat germ are also good sources. As brewer's yeast is the richest natural source, by taping a tablet between the shoulder blades, it is possible that the magnetic field of the tablet will enhance the absorption of insulin (check blood sugar levels). I have also found cabbage, spinach, peas, barley, onions and coconut to be of help in stabilizing blood sugar levels.
- **Miso:** each morning and evening.

FURTHER INFORMATION FROM THE EXPERTS

Chromium

Dr Earl Mindell (in Mindell 1988) wrote:

In the US the established, daily, safe and adequate range for this trace mineral, is between 50 and 200 mg. However, many diets only contain 25 mg per 1,000 calories. Therefore 8,000 calories per day are required to meet the upper limit of the recommendation. Since the average adult woman consumes less than 2,000 calories, it is likely that many people are deficient in this mineral. Chromium deficiency does occur and marginal chromium deficiency might be common, especially in children, women, the elderly and people who consume diets based primarily on refined foods, such as white breads and rice, frozen meals, packaged convenience foods, or other processed items. The symptoms of a chromium deficiency are closely related to the symptoms of diabetes. The first sign of deficiency is an elevation of insulin levels. The person also might feel numbness in the toes and fingers and reduced muscle co-ordination. Laboratory screening might detect elevated blood sugar levels and glucose intolerance. These symptoms are often eliminated when the person takes a chromium supplement. Chromium is also an essential factor in the regulation of cholesterol. A deficiency of this trace mineral increases a person's risk of developing atherosclerosis. In contrast, adequate intake of the mineral reduces blood cholesterol levels, and reduces a person's risk of developing heart disease. The mineral is a component of Glucose Tolerance Factor (GTF), an important substance that allows insulin to remove sugar from the blood. Without adequate amounts of chromium, and therefore GTF, insulin is secreted from the pancreas in ample amounts, but blood sugar levels remain high. This condition closely resembles the blood sugar problems noted in adult-onset diabetics. How chromium influences cholesterol levels is poorly understood. It is known, however, that as a person grows older, the likelihood of developing heart disease increases as the blood and tissue levels of chromium drop. In contrast, older people living in countries where the chromium content of the diet is high do not develop heart disease. Despite the prevalence of marginal chromium deficiencies, there are numerous excellent dietary sources of this nutrient readily available; whole-wheat bread and cereals, seafood, and Brewer's yeast. Brewer's yeast is the only dietary source of the biologically active form of chromium-GTF. This form of chromium is well absorbed and only 50 to 75 mg are needed for the body to absorb ample amounts.

Dr William Philpott of St Petersburg, Florida, a researcher with a good deal of clinical experience in treating diabetic patients, has shown a correlation between food intolerance and diabetes; when allergies have been identified, two-thirds of his patients have been able to manage their condition without insulin.

A report in 1992 stated that a slow but quite massive epidemic of childhood diabetes is emerging. In Finland, the rate had trebled since the 1950s and is increasing at the rate of 2–3% a year. Rural areas in the UK, for example Leicestershire, have experienced an 8-fold increase since the end of the Second World War. Children now take far less exercise than they used to, and this might need to be addressed if we are to stem this predicted rise. The incidence of diabetes is doubling every decade according to the medical specialists and, if this trend were to continue, then by the year 2020 nearly one-quarter of the population would be diabetic; the condition would be as common as indigestion is today (Roderick 1992).

As yet, there doesn't appear to be any sound evidence as to the causes behind diabetes and reactive hypoglycemia, other than the obvious one of defective sugar metabolism. However, defective sugar metabolism is but a symptom, with the cause of this physiological fault lying elsewhere.

Identifying the origin of physiological leaks that can eventually lead to degenerative diseases is not a mystical process. All that is required is the ability to determine the electromagnetic language of the body and react upon the information received. This is now possible and must be pursued to provide patients with the individual therapy that is their right. The lymphatic system is a mine of information that is waiting to be tapped. Vast amounts of chemicals are infiltrating our food chain, some we are told for the health of our teeth, others in order that food and drink may have a longer shelf life. Consequently, in order to maintain health and wellbeing, the need for vigilance is even greater.

The reflexology charts and acupuncture points that are relevant for the case studies in this chapter are shown in Figs 14.1 and 14.2 and are to be used in conjunction with ISR and lymphatic drainage techniques.

REFERENCES

Bergsmann O, Wooley-Hart A 1973 American Journal of Acupuncture; 1: 27–32

Burr H S 1957 Journal of Biology and Medicine; 161–167

Davies S, Stuart A 1987 Nutritional medicine. Pan Books, London

Fluoride Action Network 2000 Stop fluoride supplements for children under age 7 says Canadian Dental Association. Online. Available: http://www.fluoridealert.org

Gotzche A-L 1992 Why fluoride cannot be controlled. What Doctors Don't Tell You; 3(9): 3

Hobson J 1985 Carbohydrates: new findings could change the way you eat. Newsletter of the Hyperactivity Association of South Australia; 47: 1–5

Jones D 1999 Fluoride: damning new evidence. What Doctors Don't Tell You; 9(12): 1–4

Mindell E 1988 Chromium is necessary for life. The Vitamin Connection, 23

Mullenix P 1996 Neurotoxicity of fluoride. Fluoride; 29: 2, 57–58

Oschman J 2000 Energy medicine. Harcourt Publishers, London

Roderick D N 1992 Blood sugar control mechanisms. Enzyme Digest; April no. 6

Waldbott G L 1979 Fluoride: the great dilemma. Coronado Press, Lawrence, Kansas

Yiamouyiannis J 1999 Fluoride: damning new evidence. What Doctors Don't Tell You; 9(12)

FURTHER READING

Yiamouyiannis J 1993 Fluoride. The ageing factor. Action Press, Delaware, Ohio, pp 94–99

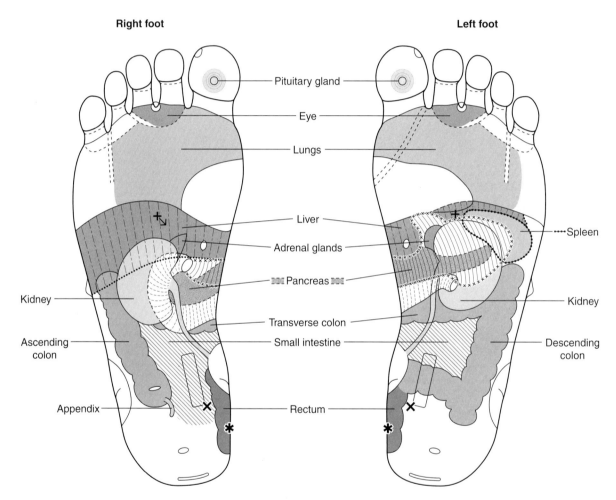

Figure 14.1 Reflexology chart for the liver, kidneys, spleen, lungs, lymph drainage points, pancreas, adrenal glands, pituitary glands, eye points, intestines and gall bladder. © F. Fox, used with permission.

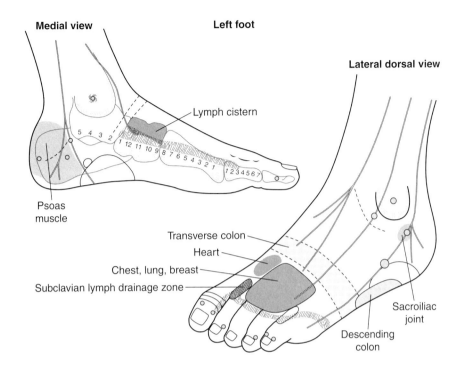

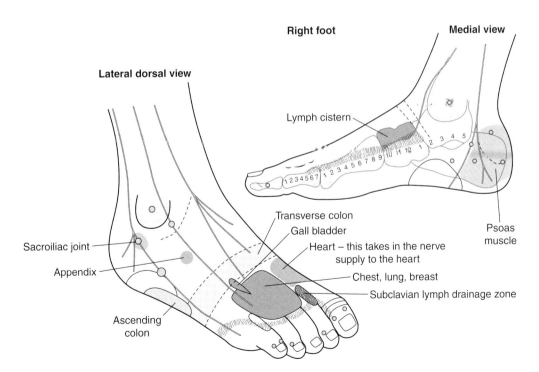

Figure 14.1 *(continued)*.

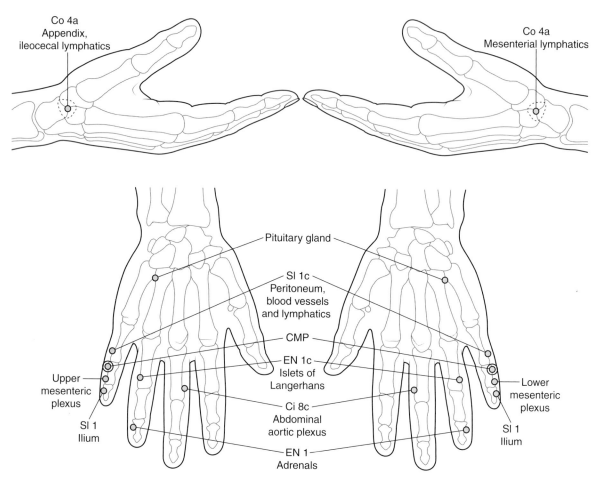

Figure 14.2 Relevant acupuncture points. The points illustrated are for fingertip testing, assessment, and acupressure only. CMP, control measurement point.

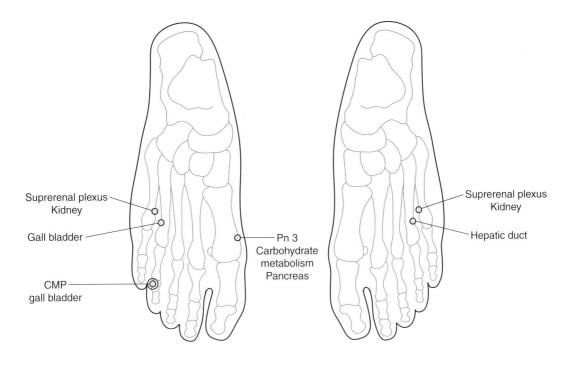

Suprerenal plexus
Kidney

Gall bladder

CMP
gall bladder

Pn 3
Carbohydrate
metabolism
Pancreas

Suprerenal plexus
Kidney

Hepatic duct

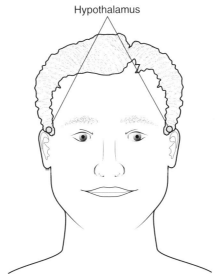

Hypothalamus

Figure 14.2 *(continued).*

15

Cobalt

About 18 years ago I had an abscess form in the gum. My dentist at that time prescribed the usual antibiotics but to no avail – the pain and swelling persisted, with the end result being tooth extraction. The missing tooth was fourth from the front, so the dentist made a denture for me. Unfortunately, the denture was very uncomfortable and I therefore did not wear it very often. A new dentist recommended a bridge. However, the drawback to this was the filing down of two healthy teeth. The prosthesis would consist of three new teeth with the outside two anchored to existing teeth.

Cobalt and dental prosthetics

Cobalt (Co) is a hard, steel–grey metallic chemical element… Cobalt blue: a dark blue pigment made from cobalt and aluminium oxides.
(Collins Pocket Dictionary)

Chrome cobalt is to be found in many dental prostheses: posts to stabilize dental crowns, bridges and the wiring used to reinforce and secure braces and dentures. It is a constituent in the coloring of some acrylate dentures (gum and palette) and fixtures. It gives metals maneuverability and so prevents breakage; for this reason it is a popular metal. This is one metal that can be visibly identified if it has permeated the tissues of the gum; the gums take on a blue hue. Cobalt is also used in stainless steel spectacles, watchbands, safety pins and paper clips. It has become apparent that this metal can often be found in bras in the underwired cups. Surprisingly, blue jeans often contain cobalt if the dye used has been made from cobalt and aluminum oxides (usually the cheaper versions) and any garments or shoes that are dark blue in color must be suspect if you want to avoid this metal.

Cobalt oxide can cause irritation to the respiratory tract, abdominal pain, nausea, vomiting, flushing of the face and ears, mild hypertension, rash and ringing in the ears. Cumulative toxic action where elimination cannot keep pace with absorption is possible. Large amounts depress erythrocyte production. Cobalt also causes irritation to skin. Symptoms include redness, itching and pain; and it might cause dermatitis. Chronic exposure, particularly oral administration, may produce goiter and reduced thyroid activity. Kidney, liver, heart and lung damage have been linked to chronic exposure of cobalt.

Aggravation of pre-existing conditions can occur in persons with skin disorders or eye problems, and people with impaired liver, kidney or respiratory function are sometimes more susceptible to the effects of cobalt. Persons with allergies or sensitivity to cobalt are also more susceptible to the effects of the substance. The website www.jtbaker.com/msds/c4961.htm provides further information on cobalt oxide.

During my training, I became aware of the dangers associated with cobalt and, as my bridge contained this metal, I discussed its removal with my dentist. However, he was rather reluctant to remove the bridge because of the vulnerability of the two teeth on either side. These teeth were capped and provided support for the bridge. It was possible that the teeth could break when the bridge was being removed leaving just the roots, and a larger gap than before. At that time there was no visible evidence of seepage into the gum above the bridge. A year later, however, I discovered the tell-tale blue hue and, within a few weeks, an abscess had formed in one of the capped teeth. Antibiotics failed to help the infection and, as a result, an apicectomy was performed. Unfortunately, this was not successful and an additional abscess formed. I consulted another dental surgeon, who performed a further apicectomy. It was at about this time that I started suffering from indigestion. Using the acupuncture points I found traces of cobalt in my stomach.

About this time, while eating a toffee, the bridge broke, severing the two supporting teeth and leaving a three-tooth gap. Until alternative materials without cobalt could be found, what was left of the teeth was cleaned, filled, and the old bridge was stuck back in place. Within a matter of weeks I started to suffer from headaches and sleepless nights, and I developed pain up into the back of my head and the side of my face. I tested myself and found cobalt. I rang my dentist and within weeks a metal was found for new posts, which were inserted into the roots of the original two teeth. The headaches and pains increased in severity and I suffered from heartburn, so I increased my treatments. I subsequently suffered tremendous pain above one of the teeth, consistent with another abscess, but an X-ray couldn't confirm this. Further dental treatment was suspended. Another apicectomy was totally out of the question and my dentist needed time to think of an alternative.

Pain in the tooth continued and pain in the stomach region increased, as did the pain up the side of my face. I was not, however, prepared for the onset of emotional disturbance that followed in the wake of the heightened symptoms. I tested the acupuncture points for the brain and found cobalt there too.

An overloading of the kidneys, spleen or liver usually causes the build-up of toxic substances in

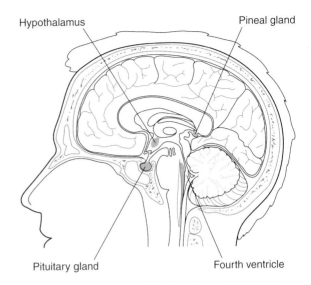

Figure 15.1 The position of the fourth ventricle, brainstem, hypothalamus, pituitary gland and pineal gland.

the brain and related organs such as the pituitary gland or the hypothalamus. However, it is possible that cobalt or mercury can enter nerve fibers in the gums and then work their way up through a cranial nerve to the brain. Most substances are prevented from entering the cerebral fluid by the blood–brain barrier, the continuous sheet of endothelial cells that lines the capillary beds and choroid plexus and which supplies cerebral fluid via the four ventricles of the brain. Water, oxygen, glucose, amino acids and lymphocytes pass quite freely through the blood–brain barrier and into the brain. Cerebral fluid circulates between the ventricles and within the fourth ventricle (cavity) of the brain. However, the barrier is absent in part of the fourth ventricle at the back of the brain (Fig. 15.1) and incomplete in other ventricles (Walton 1981, p 1291). It is therefore possible for some toxic matter to pollute the cerebral fluid and cause problems where it concentrates. Most commonly, toxic matter is trapped and forms a focus in the network of capillaries that makes up the choroid plexus or which supplies tissue fluid to the pituitary gland and the hypothalamus. One of the most vulnerable areas is the lateral ventricle on the right side of the brain. The temporal horn of the ventricle (behind the temple) lies adjacent to the hippocampus and amygdala, two parts of the limbic system. The former controls the formation of new memories and the sleep–waking cycle; the latter controls emotions such as fear, anger and sexual attraction. Sedation of the amygdala can cause docility and lack of emotional response; stimulation can cause inappropriate fear, claustrophobia, agoraphobia, anger and aggressive behavior (Barr & Kiernan 1983, pp 264–271). Another very vulnerable part of the brain is the brainstem and, closely associated with it, the pineal gland.

The brainstem

The upper portion of the brainstem is called the midbrain. On its dorsal surface are four rounded eminences called the corpora quadrigemina. These lie immediately behind the third ventricle and, if a focus forms in the choroid plexus nearby, can affect hearing and sight. Somehow this area is also connected with feelings of depression. Below the midbrain is the pons, which is connected to the cerebellum and appears to form a bridge connecting the two hemispheres of the cerebellum. However, it actually connects the cortex of each side of the brain and acts like a relay station to coordinate voluntary movements of the body. Cranial nerves VII and VIII are attached to the brainstem at the bottom end of the pons. Movements of the eyes and facial muscles, and the sense of balance and position can be affected by foci here. The bottom part of the brainstem – the medulla oblongata – is where all the other cranial nerves originate, including the vagus nerve. Foci in the medulla can cause problems with any of the cranial nerves and vital functions, and the medulla appears to be the most vulnerable part of the brainstem to disturbance by toxic substances. A focus on the cerebellum usually causes a spasm on either or both sides of the neck in the muscles where they meet the occipital ridge. This is the first area to check if problems associated with the medulla oblongata are suspected. One of the most important points to check for depression is GV 17, the acupuncture point at the back of the head on the center of the edge of the occipital ridge.

This point was aptly called 'the depression point' by Voll. I identified cobalt in this 'depression point'.

Without further delay, I had the root of the offending tooth removed. It revealed a mass of infection within the root and around the new post, which hadn't shown up on X-ray. Unfortunately, my emotional symptoms didn't clear quite so quickly. Normally I am a very positive-thinking person but I became negative, my thought pattern became sluggish and my impression of situations became distorted. My actions became almost robotic. A frightening experience occurred at the checkout in my local supermarket when I opened my purse but couldn't differentiate between the notes or coins. I panicked and could feel the palms of my hands becoming clammy. Mumbling something incoherent to the cashier I produced my credit card.

Quite alarmingly, this disruption to the brain happened very quickly once the roots of the teeth became exposed to cobalt.

The cerebral fluid is a crystal-clear, colorless liquid that fills the space between the tissues that cover the entire surface of the brain, as well as the interior of the four hollow ventricles that contain the choroid plexus. Fresh cerebral fluid extracted from the blood by the choroid plexuses and drained back into the blood mainly into the superior sagittal sinus is located in the goove between the two cerebral lobes at the top of the head. Fortunately, the material that drains out from the cerebral fluid is so fine that it rarely causes problems with the filters, although it generally comes out in sufficient quantities to be measurable by EAV testing. The blood supply for the production of cerebral fluid comes from both the vertebral arteries up the back of the neck and the internal carotid arteries in the side of the neck. The above-mentioned areas will require attention if toxic substances are to be removed from the brain.

TREATMENT

Clearing toxins from the brain can be done in a number of ways but is dependent upon the amount of toxicity and level of brain disturbance. This drainage must not be rushed and any contraindication to the actual brain drainage must be considered carefully to avoid any undue disturbance of brain waves.

The brain drain technique is an excellent complementary method for treating mental, emotional and behavioral problems. It is very safe providing the filters of the body are encouraged to function effectively for a period of time before any other steps are undertaken. See p 150 for the technique.

Full details of how to perform the exercises in the following lists are given in Appendices 1 and 2.

1. **Reflexology.** To the liver, kidneys, spleen, lungs, and lymph drainage points followed by massage above and below the clavicles (see Fig. 15.4, pp 152–153).
2. **The red light massage.**

This program must be followed by the patient for 2 weeks.

The gums are well supplied by plexuses of capillaries, including lymphatic capillaries, and any blockage of lymph in the gums and possibly the pulp will mark the beginning of an abscess. To have tone and remain pinkish in color, the gums must have a proper blood supply and free drainage; a good blood supply and venous and lymph drainage will prevent decay. The lymph must therefore be encouraged into the cervical lymph nodes, which will have been prepared for the event by the red light massage.

There are four pairs of cranial parasympathetic nerve ganglia. The submandibular ganglia each side of the lower jaw near the molar teeth are most vulnerable, and are often affected by metals from the mouth. As they control salivary production and the tension of the eardrums, they should be carefully massaged out down the neck to the drainage points.

1. **Jaw drain.** From the temporomandibular joints on both sides, massage down and under the angle of the mandible in small circular movements, working towards the center of the bone. Do this massage several times.
2. **The red light massage.**
3. **Gums.** With the pads of the fingers on the upper lips, work deep into the gums in small

circular movements. Repeat to the lower gum area, working down into the jaw.
4. From the temporomandibular joint on both sides, massage under the cheekbone, do not use undue pressure here, as this area of the skin is prone to thread veins. The patient can be encouraged to do this massage into the gum areas inside the mouth.
5. **The red light massage.**
6. Massage above and below the clavicles.
7. **Reflexology.** To the liver, kidneys, spleen, lungs, hypothalamus, pituitary gland and thyroid gland, followed by the pancreas (see Fig. 15.4, pp 152–153).

This program should be completed three times a week for 2 weeks.

Fourth week

The arachnoid villi are sponge-like structures that connect the subarachnoid space at the top of the head to the superior sagittal sinus that controls the flow of cerebral fluid into the bloodstream. They open when the pressure of cerebral fluid exceeds the venous pressure, and close when the pressure is reversed. Inverting the head causes the villi to open because it increases the pressure of the cerebral fluid.

Steps 1, 2, 3, 4 and 5 below, which achieve this pressure change, form the brain drain exercise routine.

The brain drain

Contraindications: very high blood pressure, a recent stroke and evidence of fragile capillaries.

Any patient taking medication for depression must check with their doctor before proceeding with this treatment program.

1. **Reflexology.** To the liver, kidneys, spleen, lungs, lymph drainage points, hypothalamus, pituitary gland and thyroid gland, followed by the pancreas. Massage above and below the clavicles.
2. **The red light massage.**
3. Make the patient as comfortable as possible in the prone position with the head extended well beyond the end of the table and hanging down towards the floor by 45°

(a)

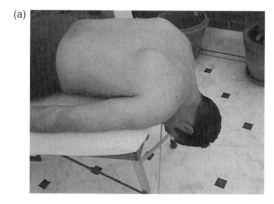

(b)

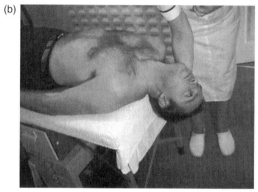

Figure 15.2 The brain drain.

(a)

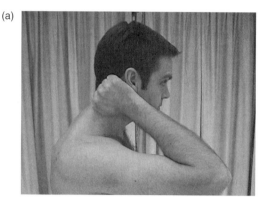

(b)

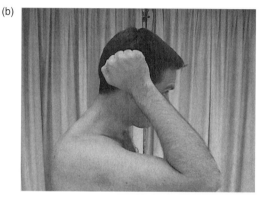

Figure 15.3 Do-in alternative to the brain drain.

(Fig. 15.2a). Maintain this position for 5 minutes.

4. Ask the patient to turn over to the supine position, with the head hanging down in the same manner for 5 minutes (Fig. 15.2b). It might be helpful to give a little reassurance at this stage by supporting the head.

5. After 5 minutes, the patient must slowly move down the table and lie horizontal for at least I minute to allow the blood pressure to stabilize.

Alternative for the patient: do-in is very successful if steps 3 and 4 are not an option.

Keep the wrist of the right hand flexed and supple and begin gentle tapping at the base of the skull just behind the right ear. Work your way gently up behind the ear over the top, and end in front of the ear to the side of the face, allowing 1-second intervals between taps. Then work backwards, starting at the temple and finishing

at the base of the skull. Repeat this procedure on the left side (Fig. 15.3).

6. The limbic lobes will need to be cleared by do-in above the top of the nose where the forehead slopes outward between the ends of the eyebrows. The limbic system consists of organs around the hypothalamus such as the amygdala and hippocampus which control mood, emotion and formation of new memories. Do-in to the area half way between the eyebrow and ear will be effective here.

7. **Exercise 1, lymph cistern.**

8. **Exercise 2, the lungs and abdomen.**

9. **Do-in.** To the bottom of the sternum and to both sides of the rib cage.

10. **Reflexology.** To the liver, kidneys, spleen, lungs, lymph drainage points, hypothalamus, pineal gland, pituitary gland, breast area and thyroid, followed by the pancreas (see Fig. 15.4). Massage above and below the clavicles.

Done correctly, this program forms the treatment for clearing the brain. This program can be repeated each week until symptoms subside. Detoxifying the brain can be a long, drawn-out process, requiring great patience and persistence. This is dependent upon the amount of toxic matter that the brain has accumulated over the years. Unfortunately, cobalt is not the only substance to stick in the brain. I find that most metals, including mercury, can adhere to the brainstem and other areas of the brain.

The patient should be advised to drink eight glasses of water a day for 3 days.

My dental treatment resumed, with a cobalt-free denture, and my depression lifted after I removed the cobalt from my brain. As often happens when a tooth has been extracted, my gum receded and the denture became loose and uncomfortable, so I resorted to a proprietary brand of denture fixative. I had used this for a week when I realized that I was not concentrating properly and I was experiencing fuzziness in my head and behind my eyes. My actions became labored and my head felt as though it was full of water. When I checked my acupuncture points I found cobalt. I originally thought it was a remnant from the bridge, until I noticed that the denture fixative was pink. I tested the fixative with the help of the snooper and discovered that it contained cobalt! I purchased a white powder that did the same job, until my gum settled down and I would be able to have another denture made. I continued to treat myself, reducing the treatments as the symptoms subsided.

I had become very aware of the emotional turbulence that I attributed to cobalt, so I was troubled when they returned yet again. Because I was watchful, the symptoms were as yet mild but I became maniacal regarding the source of this cobalt. I identified it in the cervical ganglia either side of my neck, this was one of the reasons why I had started to suffer from tight muscles in the shoulders; but I still had difficulty identifying the source, until my sister kindly offered to massage my neck and shoulders. She discovered a black line around the back of my neck. I first thought it was from the gold chain that I had been wearing, but the line was too thick. It wasn't until I went to

put my glasses back on that I realized just what had happened.

Spectacles were a new addition in my life and, to prevent the constant hunting-down of these things I had attached them to a chain to wear around my neck. The chain was a black rope design, with one of the strands gold in color. When I looked at the chain, the part that touched my neck had completely lost its gold color and had revealed a gray metal. This metal contained cobalt, and I was absorbing it through my skin.

RECOMMENDATIONS

Cobalt-free material for all dental prosthetics. This would also include the hydrated form, which is used in the making of some dentures to color the acrylate pink.

Further investigations into the absorption of cobalt into the body brought information not just as a possible cause of mental health problems but as a possible cancer risk. Cobalt is capable of traveling from the facial tissue along the stomach meridian down into the breast area, and in particular to the left breast, where it can form what is medically called a focus. A focus is a concentration of toxic matter trapped somewhere in the body with adverse consequences. Cobalt that reaches the bloodstream is filtered out by the spleen and liver. It then passes down through the bile ducts into the intestinal tract. Once it reaches the colon, it can adhere to the intestinal wall. Cobalt and its compounds have been shown to cause cancer in laboratory animals.[1]

The vast majority of bras in the shops today are underwired. If they contain cobalt it is possible that the magnetic field of the cobalt will distort nerve signal in that area, or that it is absorbed through the skin. Breast drainage exercises are explained in Chapter 7. Each female patient should be given the opportunity to take advantage of these exercises.

The reflexology charts and acupuncture points that are relevant for the case study in this chapter are shown in Figs 15.4 and 15.5 and are to be

[1] See the Material Safety Datasheet produced by jtbaker. Available: www.jtbaker.com/msds/c4961

used in conjunction with ISR and lymphatic drainage techniques.

REFERENCES

Barr M L, Kiernan J A 1983 The human nervous system. Harper & Row, New York
Walton 1981 Neurology. In: Smith L H, Thier S O (eds) Pathophysiology: The Biological Principles of Disease (International Textbook of Medicine, Vol. 1). W B Saunders, Philadelphia, p 1291

FURTHER READING

Oldfield H, Coghill R 1988 The dark side of the brain. Element Books, Dorset

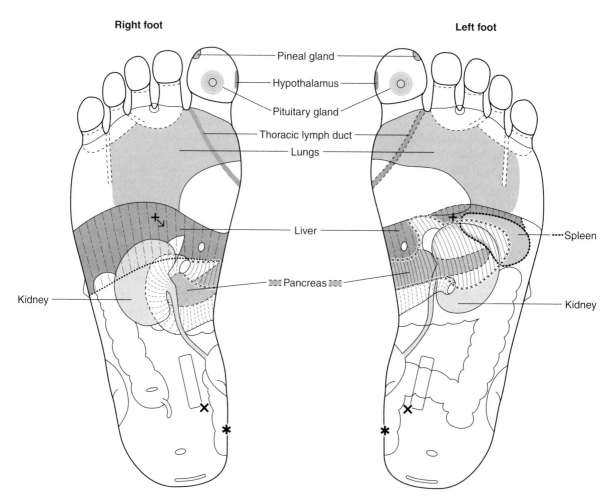

Figure 15.4 Reflexology chart for the liver, kidneys, spleen, lungs, lymph drainage points, hypothalamus, pineal gland, pituitary gland, breast area, thyroid gland and pancreas. © F. Fox, used with permission.

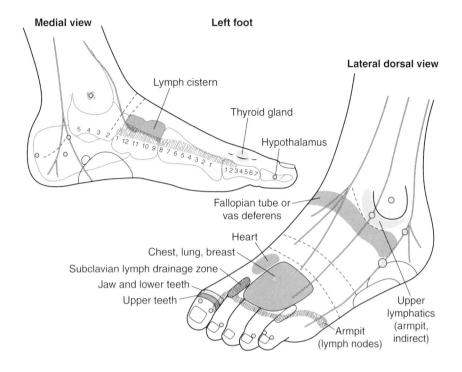

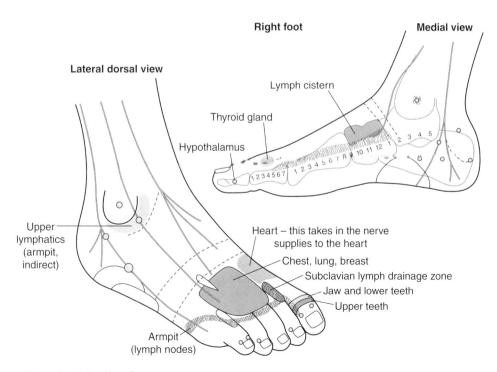

Figure 15.4 (*continued*).

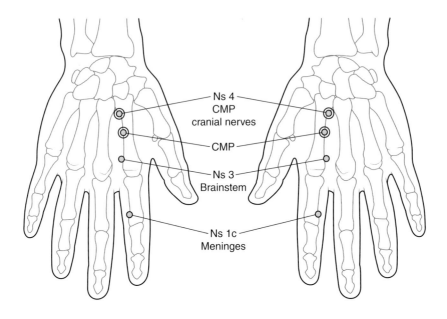

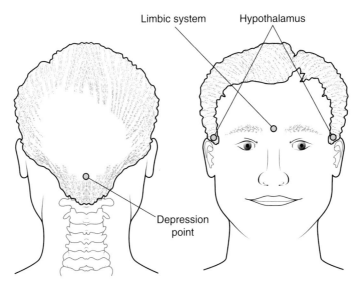

Figure 15.5 Relevant acupuncture points. The points illustrated are for fingertip testing, assessment, and acupressure only. CMP, control measurement point.

16

CASE
STUDY
11

Bad skin and hormonal imbalance

FIRST VISIT

Margaret was 38 when she first walked into the clinic. Her menstrual cycle had been irregular for some years and was now escalating, with a bleed every 10–14 days. The bleed was heavy and was accompanied by a considerable amount of pain. Breast tenderness had reached such an intensity during the last 3 months she was forced to wear a bra during the night. The burning sensation was more intense than the early days of pregnancy and, as she turned over in bed, the severe pain woke her and was seriously affecting her quality of life.

As she described the inconveniences of this condition, Margaret casually mentioned her bad acne. She felt extremely embarrassed to be suffering from this complaint at her age and it was getting worse. As a result, her doctor had prescribed tetracycline, but this was ceasing to control the condition. She was becoming increasingly concerned about her medication, one tablet a day was required 4 years before; to achieve the same results now, she had to take three.

As the interview progressed, Margaret became more eager to concentrate on her skin condition. She was so obviously distressed about her skin and she no longer felt able to talk to friends – she was hiding herself away. She felt dirty but it didn't matter how often she washed her face, nothing was helping. She thought she would be able to cope with her menstrual problems if her skin was better.

Margaret's skin was bad, particularly on her face and chest. Help had been forthcoming in the form of Betnovate (a steroid skin cream), which, although helpful for a time, made her skin thin in places. She had suffered from acne in her teens and a course of radiotherapy treatment had been prescribed. Margaret couldn't say if this form of treatment had actually improved her complexion at that time.

Margaret's medical history confirmed difficult deliveries of both her children: induced labor with her first child and a complicated home delivery with her second child, requiring emergency assistance. The complications of this second delivery eventually resulted in a prolapsed uterus.

Three years previously, at the suggestion of her GP, Margaret had consulted a gynecologist with regard to the period problems and mastitis. Replacement hormone treatment for the breast inflammation had been offered, which she refused. After the birth of her second child Margaret had suffered from phlebitis (inflammation of a vein associated with thrombosis) so her decision to refuse replacement hormone therapy was based on information linking replacement hormone involvement with thrombosis.

Hospital investigations included a laparoscopy, which revealed polycystic ovaries (although this is normally associated with scanty periods) and a large polyp on the wall of the uterus. The gynecologist explained that although the position and size of the uterus meant that the ovaries were inappropriately placed and could result in future problems, the condition was not life threatening. However, he thought a hormonal problem existed and asked her to reconsider replacement therapy. She refused once more because of her past medical history.

Margaret's acupuncture points showed that antibiotics were present in her large and small intestines, adrenal gland, hypothalamus, pituitary gland, brainstem, cervical ganglia, pancreas, liver and kidneys.

With trepidation on Margaret's part, I suggested that she replace the tetracycline with miso and vitamin and mineral supplements, provided that her doctor was in full agreement. The points for the pancreas were very congested, which suggested she was probably having some adverse reactions to certain foods. As explained in previous chapters, it is not usual to test for food sensitivities on a first visit, but this was another exception. Margaret was sensitive to: milk and its by-products, wheat, potatoes, sugar, tea and coffee. This restricted diet was to start as soon as possible.

Antibiotics

The use of antibiotics in relieving damaging infection that is threatening life or future health is of real value. Unfortunately, as so many now know, the habit of routine prescribing of these drugs for minor infections can lead to immune deficiency. The power of some drugs in fighting bacteria is phenomenal but they do not discriminate between healthy and unhealthy bacteria. Therefore, when the body is exposed to antibiotics over long periods, both directly through medication and indirectly through the consumption of meat and dairy products containing residues of antibiotics, it can cause disruption to the quality of intestinal life. Human life is only made possible through our coevolution with the bacterial world. We share an intimate union with millions upon millions of bacteria, which live both in and on us. The greatest numbers of these are housed in the intestinal tract. This mass of intestinal flora performs countless functions for the body and could be

considered as an organ in its own right. The bacteria are responsible for numerous metabolic activities, possibly even more than those of the liver, which is usually noted for its diverse action (Bryant 1987). Maintaining this healthy colony of bacteria is imperative: they clean the intestines, eliminate bad breath and flatulence, improve the complexion and assist in the health of the immune system, but they can be so easily destroyed. Antibiotics should be treated with respect and put aside for the life-threatening infections for which they are designed.

Philip Evans, a nutritionist in Colorado, is 100% convinced that most individuals feel stress and anxiety, and are prone to all sorts of ailments, because of a nutritional imbalance, but that even the best diet – one composed of all the necessary vitamins, minerals, carbohydrates, protein, etc. – will not benefit individuals nearly as much if their intestinal flora is deficient in friendly bacteria (Rowell). Without a colony of healthy bacteria, an overgrowth of the fungus *Candida* can quickly establish itself in the intestines, vagina, lungs, mouth (thrush), and on the fingernails and toenails. Hormonal changes that occur in pregnancy can also encourage growth of this fungus. This fungus – more specifically, a yeast – is usually ingested with food but can also be breathed in or picked up by contact. It seems to be almost native to the intestinal tract and appears to cause disease only when it grows out of control because of a shortage of antagonistic bacteria (healthy flora) or stagnation of the intestinal tract due to congestion of the lymphatics.

The most common and well publicized yeast is *Candida albicans*, which grows into a pathogenic form, appearing to develop a mass of threadlike filaments as it grows, which cling to the intestinal wall, putting down roots that seem capable of absorbing nourishment from the bloodstream. For this reason, it was important to consider the possibility of intestinal flora disruption and critical that Margaret introduce some form of healthy bacteria into her diet. These friendly bacteria, which are so important to our well being, can die within 5 days unless fed by milk or milk sugar (as explained in Chapter 2, when healthy bacteria are destroyed, milk intolerance will follow.) Taking miso will replenish the intestinal tract with healthy bacteria, returning it to its healthy state, which is identifiable by odorless stools.

Halting any growth of *Candida* or similar fungus is extremely important. Therefore, if there is any suspicion that either is present in a patient the following steps must be taken.

1. *Candida* appears to feed off sugars and yeast, so all foods that contain yeast must be withdrawn from the diet. Sugars in the diet should be monitored carefully.

2. Remove food and chemical sensitivities from the body and avoid unnecessary antibiotics.

3. Reflexology. To the liver, kidneys, spleen and lungs, and massage above and below the clavicles (see Fig. 16.1, p 164).

It would be advisable to repeat the above reflexology massage for 10 minutes every evening for 2 weeks.

SECOND VISIT

Margaret returned 2 weeks later and she was very distressed about her skin. There had not been the dramatic improvement she had hoped for; in fact, she thought that her skin condition had deteriorated. As her gynecological problems hadn't improved either she felt very disappointed and disheartened because she expected a miracle cure. However, she also wanted to continue with the treatment.

It was explained to Margaret that there was no quick fix to her problems. When the body has been allowed to become severely congested to this extent, the possibility of permanent damage exists.

The importance of lymphatic drainage is fundamental in the fight to combat any skin condition. The expression 'death begins in the colon' couldn't be more appropriate than in this instance. Bad skin usually manifests itself in this region – consequently, the application of many creams and lotions to the affected skin is often of no consequence because the lymphatics are congested with toxins. Without clear and nutritious tissue fluid, healthy skin is an

impossible dream. The complexion, hair and eyes reflect the health of the whole body and must not be looked at in isolation, particularly so in this case with a history of disturbed hormonal activity.

The body is balanced by circulating hormones, and the hypothalamus responds to stress, be it physical or mental. If this stress is prolonged, it can have an adverse effect on the adrenal glands and pituitary gland.

The menstrual cycle is controlled by a sequence of hormones that are produced by the hypothalamus, pituitary gland and ovaries. Any interference to this highly complex system can have an effect on hormone production. For the patient's benefit, I will explain this system further.

The endocrine system

This system consists of ductless glands, which secrete chemical messengers (hormones) directly into the bloodstream. The hormones have very specialized effects on different organs and systems of the body:

The hypothalamus

This is a prune-sized organ on the base of the brain in the middle of the head. Its cells monitor the blood and blood constituents, such as: water, minerals, glucose and hormones, and also temperature (to help the body maintain a balanced internal environment regardless of external changes). The hypothalamus sends nerve signals via the brain to the central and autonomic nervous systems via a neural stalk to the pituitary gland. It also releases hormones, which act directly or stimulate the pituitary via the portal veins and neural stalk in the infundibulum. These hormones are:

- vasopressin, to limit and thus control the amount of water excreted by the kidneys
- oxytocin, to cause contractions in the womb and release of milk in the breast in response to the baby sucking
- growth hormone releasing hormone – acts on the pituitary
- prolactin releasing factor – acts on the pituitary

- the releasing factor for the thyroid stimulating hormone – acts on the pituitary
- adrenocorticotrophic hormone releasing factor – acts on the pituitary
- the releasing factor for the follicle stimulating hormone – acts on the pituitary
- luteinizing hormone releasing factor – acts on the pituitary.

The pituitary gland

Sometimes referred to as the master gland, the pituitary is the most important of the endocrine glands because it regulates and controls the activities of other endocrine glands and many body processes. The pituitary is a pea-sized structure that hangs from the base of the brain just below the optic nerves. One of its many functions is in the development of the ovaries, and its control in the production of estrogens (British Medical Association 1990, p 804). It secretes the following hormones:

- growth hormone, to keep up the proper level of glucose in the blood
- prolactin, for the secretion of milk in the breasts
- thyroid stimulating hormone
- adrenocorticotrophic hormone, which stimulates the cortex layer of the adrenal glands to secrete corticosteroids
- follicle stimulating hormone, which acts to develop the ovaries and control the production of estrogens
- luteinizing hormone, which controls the production of progesterone.

The adrenal glands

The adrenal glands are perched on top of the kidneys and divided into two regions, the adrenal cortex and adrenal medulla.

The adrenal cortex secretes a group of hormones called corticosteroid hormones. Among its many functions are the control of blood pressure and the production of hormones that stimulate the development of male sex characteristics. It helps to produce red blood cells and acts against inflammation and allergies. After the menopause, estrogen and progesterone

production by the ovaries cease and the adrenal cortex must produce the estrogen that is still needed by the body. This is where reflexology is invaluable, as a self-help tool. Massage of the relevant points will encourage the correct secretion of estrogen.

The adrenal medulla, which is part of the sympathetic division of the autonomic nervous system, is the body's first line of defense against physical and emotional stresses. It is closely related to nervous tissue and secretes the hormones epinephrine (adrenaline) and norepinephrine (noradrenaline) in response to stimulation by sympathetic nerves. These nerves are most active during times of stress and control many of the automatic activities of the glands and organs, as in times of fight or flight.

The thyroid gland

This is found in the neck, just below the level of the larynx. The function of the gland is to make the thyroid hormones thyroxine and calcitonin, which are essential for life. These hormones control body metabolism and regulate energy levels. The secretion of these hormones is controlled by a hormonal feedback system involving the pituitary gland and hypothalamus.

The parathyroid gland is composed of four small glands embedded in the thyroid; these secrete parathormone and, it would seem, some calcitonin.

The sex glands

The testes produce testosterone in response to secretions from the pituitary gland, which is involved in the production and the development of other male characteristics.

The ovaries are a pair of almond-shaped glands situated on either side of the uterus; they produce the female sex hormones:

- estrogen – to control ovulation, the menstrual cycle, emotions and normal female sexual development
- progesterone – to prepare the womb should conception take place. If conception does not

occur, the production of progesterone drops steeply within several days, resulting in shedding of the lining of the womb and the unfertilized egg in the monthly period.

The pancreas

The islets of Langerhans are scattered throughout the pancreas and secrete insulin to facilitate the absorption of glucose.

The hormone glucagon is produced by the pancreas and needed to dissolve glycogen (glucose in storage) to provide glucose for the blood and, in emergencies, to facilitate the breakdown of protein into glucose for fuel.

Fibroids

The exact cause of fibroids is unknown, but is thought to be related to an abnormal response to estrogen hormones. Estrogen contained in oral contraceptives can cause fibroids to enlarge, as can pregnancy (British Medical Association 1990, p 447). Large fibroids can cause heavy menstrual bleeding by increasing the surface area of the uterine lining. Ovarian cysts can also produce estrogen and cause irregular vaginal bleeding (Stoppard 1994).

The endocrine system

This highly complex endocrine system usually manages its intercommunication system very well, but if the circuit of communication fails then it usually involves more than one area and can quickly activate others to overrespond in an attempt to repair the damage. The system can be compared to an orchestra, with all of the musicians playing their individual instruments in tune with the other members. Once one musician plays out of tune it will have an effect on the rest of the orchestra. Therefore, like the orchestra, any incidental change in this complicated system could develop into a more serious condition at some later stage. For this reason it would appear that to interfere unnecessarily with such a highly complex system as this is a rather foolish act.

The anatomical faults described by Margaret and confirmed by her consultant are in part the result of the action and interaction of the ductless glands. Sufficient evidence has been derived from injection of glandular extracts, from transplantation studies and from the study of diseases, to prove that these ductless glands have a profound effect on metabolism through the utilization of their secretions by other parts of the organism. How quickly, then, will the balance be disturbed by any interference to the free distribution of the lymph, which bears these secretions in its currents.

The structure and functional relations of organs with other organs regulate and assist when any breakdown that will involve the endocrine system occurs. No organ or tissue will remain normal if there is altered position in the respective regions. Perfect tone is found where vascularization and innervation remain unimpaired. Weakened ligaments allow misplacements and flexion, which will cause nodular enlargements. Varicose veins and edema can follow in many instances. A prolapsed uterus following childbirth should be dealt with in the early stages to prevent misplacement of any organs. The broad ligaments and structures will benefit enormously from abdominal massage and lymph drainage because the physiological chemistry of the body is dependent upon the state of the lymph. The vascular and lymphatic arrangement is peculiar in the pelvic basin to accommodate the changes during pregnancy. The lymph vessels are arranged so that the uterus will not obstruct them sufficiently to cause any problems. However, before any woman contemplates pregnancy there should be free drainage of the pelvic lymphatics, as this will help to prevent a prolapsed uterus after the birth, which incidentally is usually accompanied by constipation and congested pelvic lymph nodes preventing any return of lymph to the cistern. Conditions associated with hormonal imbalance must involve consideration of the hypothalamus, pituitary and the other glands of the endocrine system. However, unless the cervical lymph nodes can accommodate the lymph flow it will be useless trying to stimulate these glands to function to their optimum efficiency. The red light massage must therefore be a prominent feature in the treatment of a hormone deficiency.

Treatment

1. **Reflexology.** To the liver, kidneys, spleen, lungs, lymph drainage points, large and small intestines, adrenal gland, hypothalamus, ovaries, thyroid gland and pancreas (see Fig. 16.2, pp 166–167) followed by massage above and below the clavicle.

2. **Exercise 1, lymph cistern.** Repeat three times.

3. **Do-in.** To the base of the sternum.

4. **Abdominal massage.** Intestinal infections like *Candida* can usually be brought under control through deep, careful, massage undertaken by a trained therapist, followed by daily, morning massage by the patients themselves. Following the starvation of the *Candida* this massage encourages the now weakened threadlike filaments, to detach themselves from the intestinal wall and be carried along the digestive tract by the increased peristalsis to be processed.

5. **The red light massage.**

6. **Reflexology.** To the liver, kidneys, spleen, lungs, lymph drainage points (see Fig. 16.2, pp 166–167) and lymph cistern.

It would be advisable to repeat this program at least once a day for 2 weeks.

THIRD VISIT

Two weeks later Margaret reported many changes. Her bowel movements in particular had become regular, with a change of consistency; the usual 15 minutes spent straining hard had now ceased. Energy levels had improved; Margaret actually *wanted* to get out of bed each morning, without promising yet another early night. She suddenly became aware that this had been a long-standing problem and she was angry over the hours she had lost each day to tiredness. It took a little longer – a further 3 weeks in fact – for Margaret's skin to start

showing improvement, due in part to a sensitivity to one of her face creams. But the improvement was there and she was starting to feel hopeful.

Her menstrual problems improved slightly, as her periods became more regular and the tender breasts were less frequent. This improvement continued for 2 months until she went on holiday abroad. Unfortunately, the 9-hour plane journey appeared to affect her hormones. With only 16 days between periods, she hemorrhaged on the second day of her holiday. Luckily a doctor was on hand to reassure her that it was her menstrual flow and would ease in due course, which it did. Regretfully, on Margaret's return from holiday the tender breasts reappeared. The journey had obviously put pressure on her already struggling endocrine system, which hadn't had much of a chance to recover and upset the balance.

It was explained to Margaret that it was doubtful a solution could be found for all of her gynecological problems as quickly, if at all, to that experienced with her skin condition. Margaret had an appointment to see her gynecologist and it was discovered that the uterus was lying on the bladder and rectum. Although there were no symptoms as yet to suggest this, her gynecologist felt it was only a matter of time before problems would arise involving these organs. He suggested a hysterectomy be performed as soon as possible.

Margaret was very shocked by this news, and asked the gynecologist if she could have more time to decide. She was apprehensive about the hormone replacement implant that would be inserted during the operation to compensate for the removal of her ovaries. She wondered would this have an adverse effect on her skin, which had improved immensely, and also the possibility of thrombosis still concerned her.

Questioning both her GP and consultant on this matter was fruitless – neither could say if this was a possibility. As the left ovary was not as heavily impregnated with cysts, Margaret wanted to try and save this ovary. Her gynecologist couldn't see any reason for saving this infected organ, as it would probably need removing at some later stage anyway. The operation was scheduled for 3 month's time to allow Margaret to come to terms with the situation and for arrangements to be made for the care of her children.

Treatment

1. **Reflexology.** To the liver, kidneys, spleen, lungs, lymph drainage points, lymph cistern, fallopian tubes, pituitary gland, hypothalamus, adrenal glands and the ovaries, followed by massage above and below the clavicles.
2. **Exercise 1, lymph cistern.** Repeat three times.
3. **Abdominal massage.**
4. **Repeat Exercise 1, lymph cistern.**
5. **Do-in.** To the area just below the sternum.
6. **The red light massage.**
7. **Exercise 3, inguinal drain.** Five times each leg.
8. **Foot rotation.**
9. **Repeat Exercise 1, lymph cistern.**
10. **Exercise 8, the islets of Langerhans and the carbohydrate function of the pancreas.**
11. **Exercise 9, the deep inguinal nodes.**
12. **Repeat Exercise 1, the lymph cistern.**
13. **Do-in.** As in brain drain (p 150).
14. **The red light massage.**
15. **Do-in.** To the base of the sternum.
16. **Reflexology.** To the liver, kidneys, spleen, lungs, lymph drainage points, lymph cistern, fallopian tubes, pituitary gland, hypothalamus, adrenal glands and the ovaries, followed by massage above and below the clavicles.

It would be advisable for the patient to repeat this program twice a week for 2 weeks, although reflexology should be performed each evening. However, the patient should be seen on a weekly basis for 1 month to ensure that abdominal massage and the drainage steps are done professionally. Back and neck massage working deep into the occipital ridge can be a consideration for the therapist to incorporate within the treatment program and the following steps can be introduced during this period. These can form part of the patient's alternative treatment program:

1. **Reflexology.** To the liver, kidneys, spleen, lungs, lymph drainage points, lymph cistern, fallopian tubes, pituitary gland, hypothalamus, adrenal glands and the ovaries, followed by massage above and below the clavicles.
2. **Exercise 1, lymph cistern.** Repeat three times.
3. **Abdominal massage.**
4. **Repeat Exercise 1, lymph cistern.**
5. **Do-in.** To the area just below the sternum.
6. **Exercise 10, thyroid and parathyroid lymph nodes.**
7. **Exercise 6, the brainstem.**
8. **Exercise 2, lungs and upper abdomen.**
9. **Do-in.** To the base of the sternum then proceed up the sternum then to the sides of the rib cage.
10. **Reflexology.** To the liver, kidneys, spleen, lungs, lymph drainage points, lymph cistern, fallopian tubes, pituitary gland, hypothalamus, adrenal glands and the ovaries, followed by massage above and below the clavicles.

The above two treatment programs must never be completed at any one-treatment session. Rather, the steps should be alternated, providing the filters are functioning effectively.

The charts Margaret took home to guide her on the zones for reflexology remained virtually unchanged. She became meticulous regarding every detail of the home treatment program. Each time her acupuncture points were tested they showed an improvement and her body was eventually becoming clear. Although she still suffered from tender breasts before her periods this appeared to be a normal monthly hormonal response. The significant improvement was to her skin. Margaret's conscientiousness increased and she began to massage the points on the feet for the ovaries twice a day. She was obviously torn between how much time to give reflexology, and the situation inside her pelvis. With minor adjustments to her chart and diet, her health improved tremendously. No longer was she catching colds from the children – a sore throat was now a thing of the past and minor cuts healed so quickly. A feeling of wellbeing was how Margaret described her emotional state: her new-found clear skin was giving her more and more confidence. I questioned Margaret about her sore throats. Apparently, from an early age she had suffered on a regular basis from tonsillitis and from recollection she had received antibiotics almost every 3 months for the condition! This was probably one of the reasons why the cervical ganglia were so congested and her neck muscles were so rigid.

After 3 months, Margaret underwent surgery, feeling that she couldn't be in better health to face major surgery. Two days after her operation she phoned, sounding very excited. Although certain problems had presented themselves during the operation, this was due in the main to her very enlarged uterus adhering to other organs, which prolonged the surgical procedure. The surgeon, however, had decided to leave her left ovary, as it was free from cysts. Not wanting to change any pattern in her diet, Margaret had arranged for her special food to be brought into the hospital.

Two months after her operation Margaret looked in good health. Her clear skin had improved her confidence and her diet had provided boundless energy. She was fortunate that scarring of her skin due to the pustules had been minimal and was becoming less visible.

Margaret continued with her diet, but was able to reintroduce foods previously banned after about 12 months. The occasional cups of coffee and tea, and small amounts of chocolate, appeared not to affect her skin. It seemed inevitable that she would never be able to tolerate white bread or cream and cheese. If a small amount of cheese was ever eaten, her face responded with at least one spot the next day. The health of her family also improved after they started receiving reflexology from Margaret.

Because Margaret's gynecologist is adamant that her left ovary will eventually have to be removed, she is meticulous in her reflexology and lymph drainage exercises. Regular pelvic scans have not revealed any abnormality to the left ovary. As her hysterectomy was 15 years ago she is hopeful that she will go through the menopause normally without any more trouble.

Medical treatment

I must draw to the attention of therapist and patient the following passage:

Surgical removal of ovarian cysts is always required, whatever the type of ovarian cyst, as only microscopic examination of the cyst distinguishes a malignant tumour from a benign one. The likelihood of the cyst being cancerous increases as you get older. (Stoppard 1994)

For this reason, the medical profession must be consulted if there is any suspicion regarding an ovarian cyst, to necessitate the relevant treatment.

Patient guide

The following were successfully used as part of Margaret's rehabilitation program (consult your GP before taking any supplements):

- Water: it is advisable to drink eight glasses of water a day for 3 days after intense lymphatic drainage therapy.
- Any patient suffering from prolonged skin problems should be advised to have a blood/urine test for diabetes.
- Vitamin E: 400 iu daily.
- Vitamin C: 1 g daily (required by the adrenal glands to absorb the raw materials for the production of their hormones).
- Yeast-free vitamin B complex: one daily.
- Zinc: one daily.
- Dolomite: three daily (this is magnesium and calcium) if this is not available take 100 mg of magnesium daily.
- Multivitamin and mineral: one daily.
- Evening primrose oil: 1000 mg daily.
- Nettle tea: two cups daily. *Caution*: the suitability should be checked in patients suffering from hypertension.
- Green tea: at least two cups daily.
- New Era Tissue Salts: kali phos for low energy.
- New Era Tissue Salts: kali sulph, which helps with all skin problems.
- Echinacea: to support the immune system. Take one capsule a day for 2 weeks in every 2-month period (do not take if pregnant).
- Bach Flower Remedies: The first remedies that Margaret responded to were Crab Apple,

Cerato and Wild Rose. She took this combination for 1 month. Walnut followed. Margaret responded extremely well to this remedy, which she took for 1 month, and then as and when she felt in the need of its support.

- Miso: twice daily. An amount the size of the small fingernail is to be taken each evening before going to bed and half an hour before breakfast the following morning. *Note*: do not take miso with hot water.

   Japanese Miso is unpasteurized fermented soybean, rice or barley purée. It is a known fact that Japanese women seldom suffer from menopausal symptoms; this could be as a direct result of taking miso.

- Estrogen-like hormones known as phytoestrols, can be found in rhubarb, all soya products, celery, fennel, ginseng, liquorice and nettle.

REFLEXOLOGY

Estrogen and progesterone production by the ovaries ceases during the menopause. The onus falls on to the adrenal cortex, which must produce the estrogen still needed by the body. Reflexology can be of enormous assistance during this transitional period and the final chart will suffice for this purpose.

THE SECRET OF BEAUTIFUL SKIN

The lymphatics of the face are just as likely to be congested as any other part of the body. Expensive creams and lotions applied to the skin can cause as much congestion and damage as elsewhere in the body and many do contain chemicals. Before a chemical can cause a toxic response in the skin, or indeed anywhere else in the body, it must first penetrate the skin's major barrier and outermost layer. The chemical must then enter the living epidermis and it is here that toxicity can start, as the skin responds adversely,

leading to dermatitis, acne or cancer. The toxin then reaches the upper dermis, which consists of connective tissue, lymphocytes, nerves, blood vessels and lymphatics, and finally it enters the general circulation, to be carried to distant sites (Hotchkiss 1994). Margaret is testimony to the remarkable change in skin condition that can be achieved by correct diet and lymphatic drainage.

Face drainage

1. **Red light massage** (Appendix 2, p 184).

2. With a little oil on the fingers, place the index finger and thumb of both hands behind the ears so that each ear sits in the base of the index finger and middle finger (Fig. 16.1a).

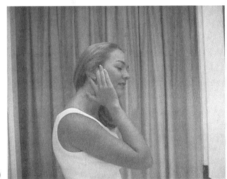

16.1(a)

3. Pull both hands firmly down the side of the face (Fig. 16.1b). Do this ten times.

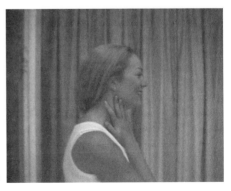

16.1(b)

4. Place each thumb just below the ear and under the jawbone (Fig. 16.1c). Gently massage the space behind the jawbone, moving as you do towards the chin and finishing up with both thumbs just underneath the chin (Fig. 16.1d). Do this ten times.

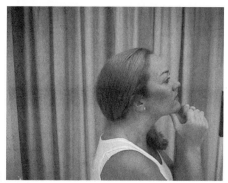

16.1(c)

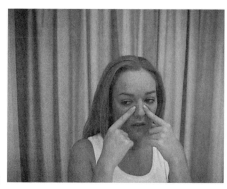

16.1(d)

5. Place each index finger either side of the bridge of the nose and massage in a circular motion down and under the cheekbones to the ears (Fig. 16.1e, f). *Note*: be careful about the amount of pressure you use in this area if you are prone to thread veins. Do this ten times.

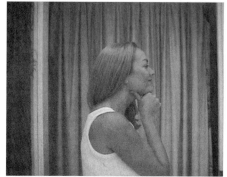

16.1(e)

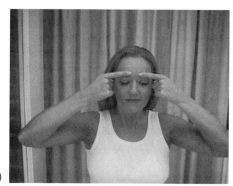

16.1(f)

6. Place each index finger atop of the eyebrows and massage in a circular motion down towards each ear (Fig. 16.1g). Do this ten times.

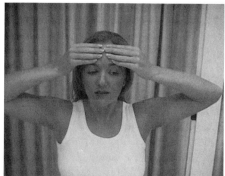

16.1(g)

7. With the pads of your fingers placed in the center of the forehead (Fig. 16.1h) massage from the center out and down towards the ears. Do this ten times.

16.1(h)

8. Repeat step 2.
9. Repeat the red light massage and massage above and below the clavicles.

Performing Exercise 6 after this face massage clears all of the lymph nodes that drain the scalp, face and external ear.

Face massage is to be avoided in the presence of pustules.

The following tests are to be used as a guide. The patient is advised to consult their doctor if a problem is suspected.

Adrenal gland test

The following procedure will give an instant assessment of adrenal efficiency. Blood pressure should be taken while lying down for 4 minutes. It is then taken again immediately on standing up. If the higher of the two figures recorded is not at least five points higher when standing, as compared to lying down, then the adrenals are considered to be underfunctioning.

Thyroid gland test

This test is based on the Barnes basal temperature test. It should be used as a guide only. Supplementing the diet with kelp will, in many cases, improve thyroid function.

The underarm temperature is recorded on three successive mornings before getting up and before any food or drink has been consumed. The thermometer is left in position for 10 minutes and the three recordings are written down. Calculate the average of the three recordings.

Women who have not ceased menstruation should take the readings starting on the second day of their period. If the result is an average below 97.8°F (36.6°C) then the thyroid can be considered to be underactive. If the average is above 98.2°F (36.8°C) then the thyroid can be considered to be overactive. An overactive thyroid can lead to exhaustion (What Doctors Don't Tell you 1996).

The 'reflexology charts' and acupuncture points that are relevant for this case study are shown in Figs 16.2 and 16.3 and are to be used in conjunction with ISR and lymphatic drainage techniques.

REFERENCES

British Medical Association 1990 Complete family health encyclopaedia. Dorling Kindersley, London
Bryant M 1987 Probiotics – a new direction in medicine. Felmore Health Publications: number 137
Hotchkiss S 1994 How thin is your skin? New Scientist; 26: 24–27
Rowell D What *Acidophilus* does. Felmore Health Publications: number 31
Stoppard M 1994 Menopause. London, Dorling Kindersley, p 99
What Doctors Don't Tell You 1996; 6(7): 8

FURTHER READING

Berg R 1983 Human intestinal microflora in health and disease. Academic Press, London
Draser B S, Hill M J 1984 Human intestinal flora. Academic Press, London

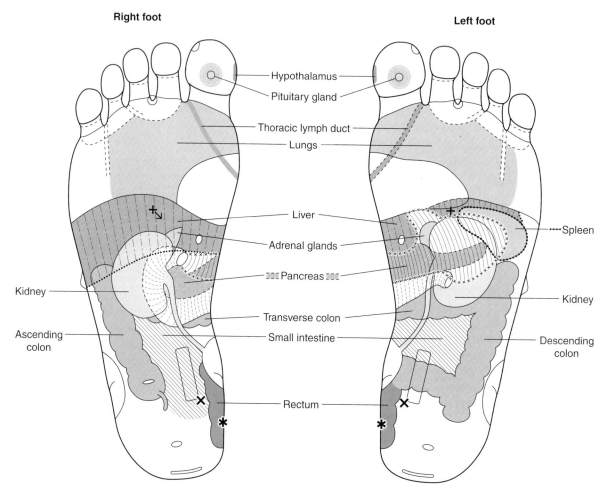

Right foot

Left foot

- Hypothalamus
- Pituitary gland
- Thoracic lymph duct
- Lungs
- Liver
- Spleen
- Adrenal glands
- Pancreas
- Kidney
- Kidney
- Transverse colon
- Ascending colon
- Small intestine
- Descending colon
- Rectum

Figure 16.2 Reflexology chart for the liver, kidneys, spleen, lungs, lymph drainage points, large and small intestines, adrenal gland, fallopian tubes, pituitary gland, hypothalamus, ovaries, thyroid gland and pancreas. © F. Fox, used with permission.

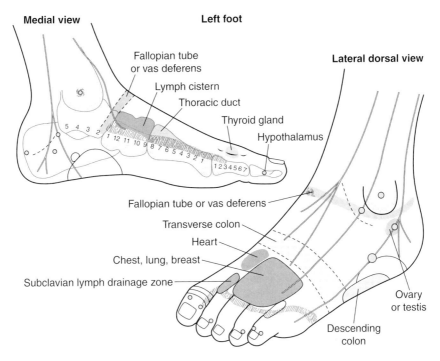

Figure 16.2   (*continued*). Unless otherwise stated, all reflex zones apply to both feet.

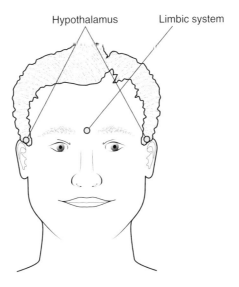

Figure 16.3

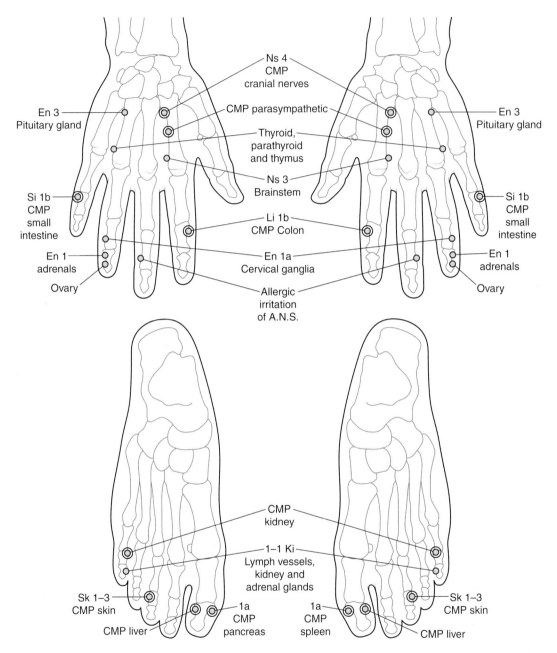

Figure 16.3 (*continued*). Relevant acupuncture points. The points illustrated are for fingertip testing, assessment, and acupressure only. CMP, control measurement point.

17

Let the body choose

My purpose in this book has been to show the relationship between degenerative disease and physiological faults in the body and to suggest ways in which they can be replaced by good health. Nature did not intend that we should be bombarded with excessive amounts of chemicals or metals and therefore the body is ill-equipped to tolerate them in any form. These substances can go undetected for years, masquerading as bloatedness, tiredness, migraine, backache, headache, obesity and many other irritating symptoms, until the body succumbs to their assaults and deteriorating health ensues. The human body is seen by Western medicine as a perfunctory machine, whose mechanisms can be learned, understood and serviced by a mechanic. The emphasis is on diagnosing and treating illness rather than preventing it. Unfortunately, this individual matrix of organs and cells is not a vintage car and cannot be repaired by following a procedure in a mechanics' manual on diagnosis and repair. Quite the contrary, the human body is unique to the individual, whose wants and needs are constantly changed by the demands of modern civilization. But science is not equipped to cope with individual requirements. Drugs are administered en mass in the hope that all individuals will respond in a way that can be anticipated and predetermined. However, as individuals we respond specifically.

The emphasis throughout this book is on the forgotten ability of individuals to participate in the care of their health. We each possess a unique ability and power to identify not only any physiological faults that exist within but also the substances that are responsible for or likely to cause those faults. The goal is to discover ways by which any problem can be dealt with in its very early stages and thereby prevent degenerative disease.

Is this possible? Yes – but the responsibility is a combined one.

Taking responsibility for and participating in the prevention of serious illness will reduce the need for curative interventions. Patient participation and the ability to decide what is right for the body, rather than being dependent on advice that can be contradictory and confusing, is the right of the individual. An old Chinese proverb says: 'Give a man a fish and you feed him for a day. Teach him how to fish and you feed him for a lifetime'.

I am not suggesting that modern medical treatment should be forsaken, rather, that both forms of therapy be combined. With about 340 acupuncture points on the hands and feet alone to choose from and all of them vibrating with vital information about the physiological health of the body, it is inconceivable that such a comprehensive form of investigation and treatment is not fully utilized.

ISR, in its uniqueness of application combined with lymphatic drainage exercises, sets this therapy apart from any other. Nature has provided this knowledge and its many advantages will be appreciated.

The information has been presented in a format that provides the therapist and patient with an understanding of the therapy and, through the case studies, examples of how the body is capable of helping itself. I feel confident that the discovery and experience will enable life to be lived to the full and retirement will be full of the enjoyment of the pleasures that a long and pain-free existence will provide.

SECTION 3

Appendices

SECTION CONTENTS

Therapist exercises

CONTRAINDICATIONS FOR DEEP LYMPH DRAINAGE EXERCISES

1. **Overloading of the liver, kidneys, spleen and lungs with toxins or toxic amounts of any substance.** However, if such overloading is due to toxins already in lymph nodes near the autonomic ganglia and plexus that control these organs, those substances must first be moved prior to any further drainage. The filters should then be allowed to deal with these substances before more material is transported to them for filtration. In addition, congestion of the lymph stream at the emptying point of the thoracic duct and right lymphatic duct from possible tension in the muscles of the area will need to be addressed before any lymphatic drainage can begin. For this reason, massage to the area above and below the clavicles and reflexology to stimulate the filters is needed prior to any lymph drainage exercises.

2. **Infectious diseases with raised temperature.** The lymphatics should be given time to bring such infections under control and break down the affected matter. Infected matter should never be forced into the bloodstream prematurely because of the risk of blood poisoning.

3. **Acute inflammation or fever caused by poisons, bacteria or viruses.** Again, because of the danger of blood poisoning, phagocytosis and chelation (binding with protein, especially albumin) should be allowed to take place first.

4. **Varicose veins.** Massage of the legs is contraindicated, although the lymphatics should be cleared, as congestion could be restricting venous flow, for example the superficial and deep inguinal nodes. It is wiser to work on the efferents to assist lymph drainage rather than over the actual nodes and abdominal massage could certainly be beneficial. Massage to the reflex zones of the legs should be undertaken.

5. **Asthma.** Lymph drainage exercises should not be performed during an asthmatic attack.

6. **Cardiac edema.** However, reflexology is not contraindicated for the above conditions.

7. **Recent thrombosis or evidence of fragile capillaries (e.g. constant nose bleeds).**

8. **Cancer** (see Chapter 5).

9. **For brain drain.** Very high blood pressure, a recent stroke, evidence of fragile capillaries.

10. **Brittle bones.**

As the majority of exercises are performed by the patient under the guidance of the therapist, all the relevant photographs are included in Appendix 2.

EXERCISE TECHNIQUES

EXERCISE 1, LYMPH CISTERN

Place one hand over the abdomen by the navel and ask the patient to push-out the abdomen against your hands without breathing in. The patient should inhale deeply while maintaining the pressure against your hands, even increasing it for a short time before relaxing and exhaling. Repeat three times.

You must make sure that the pressure exerted is directed to the hands on the navel; the patient must not direct any pressure to the head.

EXERCISE 2, LUNGS AND UPPER ABDOMEN

Caution: if there is a problem with brittle bones, the patient must not put pressure on the ribs, but direct the breath towards the hands.

Crossing the arms in front of the body and placing the hands over the lower rib cage on each side, the patient needs to take a deep breath. While holding the breath, and without putting any pressure into the head, the breath should be directed towards the hands while exerting a little pressure on the sides of the rib cage. Repeat three times.

To ensure that filtrate from the root of the lungs enters the lymph cistern, massage from the edge of the rib cage in line with the nipple down towards the navel.

Do this exercise three times on each side.

Alternative to Exercise 2

In the event that Exercise 2 proves difficult for young children and the elderly, revert to this alternative. Do-in to the lymph nodes under the intercostal spaces both in the front and to the back of the rib cage. Tapping gently, move up and down the rib cage back and front.

EXERCISE 3, INGUINAL DRAIN

This exercise clears the lymphatics of the small intestine, colon and the area around the rectum, and reduces any spasm that forms in the psoas muscles.

With the patient in the supine position, place a rolled, medium-sized hand towel in the right groin and instruct the patient to bend the right leg and, holding the knee, pull it up towards the chest with both hands. Hold it there for about 10 seconds to allow the lymph to drain up into the lymph cistern. Then repeat the exercise with the left leg. This procedure should be repeated four more times.

FOOT ROTATION

This exercise stimulates the muscles of the thigh and activates the nerves, which supply energy to the muscles and ligaments of the pelvis. This helps to release any compression on the sciatic nerve and, combined with Exercise 3, is very successful for pelvic and lower back conditions.

With the patient supine and the right leg raised about 6 inches off the treatment couch, rotate the raised foot by the ankle ten times one way and ten times the other. Repeat with the left leg. Then ask the patient to perform this exercise themselves, asking him or her to draw a circle in the air with the big toe.

When this exercise is first performed the rotating foot will possibly shudder as it moves around, not quite forming a circle. As the nerve supplies in the pelvic region improve so too will the ability of the patient to draw a perfect circle in the air with both feet. This outward sign signals the regeneration of interconnecting energy fields and repair. Ideally this exercise should be carried out at home morning and evening. But, to a lesser degree, just rotating the ankles while sitting at a desk, at traffic lights or watching the television will help enormously in keeping the energy fields vibrating.

Together, these exercises combined with reflexology, lymph drainage point massage, Exercise 1 and do-in, would be beneficial before any long-haul flight. Foot rotation could then continue during the flight at half-hour intervals.

EXERCISE 4, THE FOUR-STEP EXERCISE

This helps to stimulate the nerve supplies of the celiac plexus, abdominal aortic plexus, solar plexus, duodenum and jejunum and decongests the superior mesenteric lymph nodes in the epigastrium. It is best performed by the patient under the guidance of the therapist but can be repeated at home.

1. **Step one:** with the tip of the right thumb at the base of the sternum, press the heel of the thumb down deep along the right edge of the rib cage. The patient must exert abdominal pressure against the thumb several times for about 5 seconds. This forces the lymph into the lymph cistern, which must be cleared prior to further lymph drainage exercises.

2. **Step two:** Exercise 1, lymph cistern.

3. **Step three:** repeat step one but on the left edge of the rib cage.

4. **Step four:** repeat Exercise 1, lymph cistern.

EXERCISE 5, THE BRONCHIAL PLEXUS

The bronchial plexus is on the artery supplying the bronchi and bronchiole, and lies behind the sternum on the 3rd sternal groove. Stimulation of this plexus is achieved by clearing the lymphatics behind the sternum using a simple massage:

1. Massage firmly with the fingertips along the third depression of the sternum for a few minutes then, moving down to the fourth depression, repeat the exercise to clear the bronchial lymph nodes.

2. Massage up along each side of the sternum. This helps to keep the parasternal lymph nodes clear too.

If this massage technique is part of a maintenance program for people with asthma, it is very important that the exercise is not repeated more than once during each treatment session. It is wiser, when treating these patients, to progress slowly. This allows for the lungs to adjust to the level of carbon dioxide from the blood, which is increased once the functions of the lungs improve. This is a massage that some women might prefer to be accomplished in partnership with the therapist.

Clearance of the lungs and heart can be checked on NS 2 on the epicondyle at the base of the index finger lateral side.

EXERCISE 6, THE BRAINSTEM

The therapist will be familiar with the massage technique that is required.

1. Insert the thumbs of both hands underneath the occipital bone at its center point and massage into the ridge.

2. Follow the line of the ridge and work into the mastoid process for about 3 minutes with the thumbs.

3. Massage across and down the neck either side of the vertebral arteries to assist in the interconnection of energy between the medulla oblongata, the pons and the midbrain, as deeply as is comfortable for the patient.

EXERCISE 7, LYMPH DRAINAGE OF THE HEART

Note: This exercise should be performed only after Exercises 2, 5 and 6, and never on its own.

The deepest lymph nodes lie just behind the 5th intercostal spaces on each side of the sternum, and out as far as below each nipple. The lymph from the left side drains under the sternum to the lymph nodes next to the sternum on the right. Lymph from the right side drains into the same area and then, together, up through the lymphatics to the lymphatic duct. Massage with the fingertips along the route of drainage. It should be noted that the lymphatics of the endocardium and myocardium drain into the nodes to the left of the sternum, while those of the pericardium drain into the nodes to the right of the sternum. When this massage has been completed ask the patient to take a deep breath and hold it while you position the palm of your hand against the epigastrium. Press gently but firmly towards the heart, at the same time ask the patient to push the diaphragm out against the palm of your hand while holding the breath. You should feel this pressure against your hand, hold this position for 6 seconds before asking the patient to relax. It is important that the patient does not exert pressure to the head during this exercise, rather, direct it towards your hand. Repeat this exercise three more times. Eventually you might hear a little gurgle in the small intestine or colon, or feel a slight movement in the epigastrium. As the lymph drainage of the heart clears, a spurt of energy goes to the small intestine.

EXERCISE 8, TO CLEAR THE NERVE SUPPLY TO THE ISLETS OF LANGERHANS AND THE CARBOHYDRATE FUNCTION OF THE PANCREAS

Roll up a medium-sized hand towel, place it in the right groin and then, either sitting or lying, ask the patient to bend the right leg by the knee and pull it up towards the chest with both hands. Hold it there for about 10 seconds to allow the lymph to drain up into the lymph cistern. While in this position, the patient must push out the abdomen against the towel and breathe in deeply. Repeat the exercise with the left leg. This procedure should be repeated four more times.

EXERCISE 9, THE DEEP INGUINAL NODES

Exercises 8 and 9 can be of benefit where frequent urination is a problem and can enhance performance of the organs in the lower abdomen.

Note: A therapist carrying out this procedure must use the hypothenar eminence and should ask the patient's permission before any physical therapy to this sensitive area. The exercise can be performed over light clothing.

While exerting pressure that is comfortable to the patient in the area of the horizontal group of inguinal lymph nodes on the right side, ask the patient to draw in the lower abdomen, as if to suck up the lymph from that area. Repeat twice more before carrying out the procedure on the left group of nodes.

EXERCISE 10, THYROID AND PARATHYROID LYMPH NODES

The patient under the guidance of the therapist best performs this exercise:

1. Massage deep into the tissues above and below the clavicle several times, spending some time on the lymph drainage points.

2. Massage deep into the acromioclavicular joint.
3. Perform the red light massage.
4. Place the left hand over the throat, with the thumb and middle finger resting just under the base of the jaw. Massage down either side of the larynx and out along the clavicle above and below. Do exactly the same with the other hand.

ABDOMINAL MASSAGE

This abdominal massage has been perfected over many years in conjunction with EAV and ISR. Having the facility to measure the improvement to energy fields produced by this physical therapy was fascinating.

Begin by gently palpating the abdomen to relax the patient, who might feel discomfort due to congested lymph nodes. As the muscles relax, the therapist can start to massage, being aware of areas of sensitivity.

Proceed to gently massage, with small circular movements, in the region of the ascending colon in a clockwise direction. Work towards the hepatic flexure, concentrating on this area for several minutes moving on across the transverse colon into the splenic flexure, again concentrating here for several minutes. This process must continue until the tissue feels relaxed. At this stage, the pressure of massage should deepen, whereupon concentration is focused on the appendix/cecal area, working into and under the anterior superior iliac spine for some minutes, provided the patient does not feel any discomfort. Continue in this vein while moving up through the colon and over to the left side and down into the sigmoid colon, where massage will continue for a few minutes. At this stage move to the region of the small intestine and continue with small circular movements again for a few minutes. Persist in this method for approximately 20 minutes.

THE RED LIGHT MASSAGE

This exercise clears the cervical lymph nodes permitting the cervical ganglia to function to their optimum ability. It is so called because massaging the sides of the neck can easily be done while sitting at traffic lights. As the thyroid and parathyroid glands depend upon nerve impulses from the cervical ganglia, it would be most beneficial for this exercise to become a daily activity for the prevention of other conditions for all patients. For instance, hypothyroidism (which causes tiredness and can contribute to obesity), hyperthyroidism (which can lead to weight loss) and osteoarthritis and osteoporosis (which are due to faulty calcium metabolism), can all benefit from this massage. As the heart and lungs can also benefit from the energetic interaction that is encouraged by this massage, it can pay dividends to be rigorous in its application. It will, however, take about 3 weeks for the nerve impulses from the ganglia to return to normal.

With the flat of the fingers, press quite firmly from just beneath the mastoid process down the sternocleidomastoid and into the scalenus mediaus, ending in the acromioclavicular joint each side. Repeat this 15 times.

THE ROWING BOAT EXERCISE

The therapist should supervise this exercise.

This exercise can be a bit difficult at first but is beneficial in helping to improve the nerve supply and tone to the muscles of the neck and upper spine.

1. Ask the patient to sit on a stool in front of a mirror. The back should be straight; imagine a book is balancing on the head.

2. The patient hunches the shoulders so that the neck disappears and the base of the skull can be felt touching the top of the spine.

3. The patient bends the elbows and brings the arms, with clenched fists, level with the chest.

4. Finally, the patient slowly and deliberately pushes the elbows back, at the same time forcing the chest forwards, and brings the head out from its sunken position as though the head is being pulled upwards and the shoulders are about to touch each other behind the back.

5. The patient finishes by placing the hands, palm-side up, one on top of the other in the lap to relax the muscles, taking slow breaths for a couple of seconds, before repeating the process.

This exercise should be repeated five times each morning and evening to encourage lymphatic drainage in the neck and shoulder region.

Other techniques are described in the relevant chapters:

- breast drain (see Chapter 7)
- stomach wash (see Chapter 10 and Appendix 2)
- blood pressure (see Chapter 13)
- the brain drain (see Chapter 15)
- gall bladder (see Appendix 2)
- thymus (see Appendix 2).

Appendix 2

Patient exercises

CONTRAINDICATIONS FOR DEEP LYMPH DRAINAGE EXERCISES

1. **Overloading of the liver, kidneys, spleen and lungs with toxins or toxic amounts of any substance.** However, if such overloading is due to toxins already in lymph nodes near the autonomic ganglia and plexus that control these organs, those substances must first be moved prior to any further drainage. The filters should then be allowed to deal with these substances before more material is transported to them for filtration. In addition, congestion of the lymph stream at the emptying point of the thoracic duct and right lymphatic duct from possible tension in the muscles of the area will need to be addressed before any lymphatic drainage can begin. For this reason, massage to the area above and below the clavicles and reflexology to stimulate the filters is needed prior to any lymph drainage exercises.

2. **Infectious diseases with raised temperature.** The lymphatics should be given time to bring such infections under control and break down the affected matter. Infected matter should never be forced into the bloodstream prematurely because of the risk of blood poisoning.

3. **Acute inflammation or fever caused by poisons, bacteria or viruses.** Again, because of the danger of blood poisoning, phagocytosis and chelation (binding with protein, especially albumin) should be allowed to take place first.

4. **Varicose veins.** Massage of the legs is contraindicated, although the lymphatics should be cleared, as congestion could be restricting venous flow, for example the superficial and deep inguinal nodes. It is wiser to work on the efferents to assist lymph drainage rather than over the actual nodes and abdominal massage could certainly be beneficial. Massage to the reflex zones of the legs should be undertaken.

5. **Asthma.** Lymph drainage exercises should not be performed during an asthmatic attack.

6. **Cardiac edema.**

However, reflexology is not contraindicated for the above conditions.

7. **Recent thrombosis or evidence of fragile capillaries (constant nose bleeds).**

8. **Cancer** (see Chapter 5).

9. **For brain drain.** Very high blood pressure, a recent stroke, evidence of fragile capillaries.

10. **Brittle bones.**

EXERCISE TECHNIQUES

EXERCISE 1, LYMPH CISTERN
(Fig. A2.1)

Place both hands over the abdomen by the navel and push-out the abdomen against the hands without breathing in. Take a deep breath while maintaining pressure to the hands, and even increasing the pressure for a short time before relaxing and exhaling.

(a)
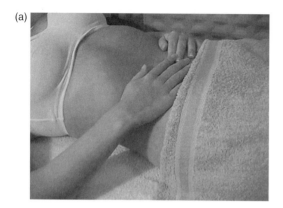

(b)
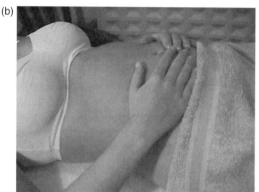

Figure A2.1   Exercise 1: lymph cistern. (a) Preparation for Exercise 1; (b) performing the exercise.

(a)
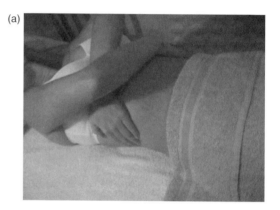

(b)
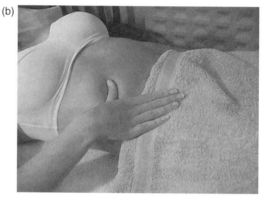

Figure A2.2   Exercise 2: lungs and upper abdomen and filtration of the lung entering the cistern.

Do not put any pressure into the head. Rather, direct it towards the navel otherwise the lymph cistern will not clear. Repeat three times.

EXERCISE 2, LUNGS AND UPPER ABDOMEN (Fig. A2.2)

Caution: do not put pressure on the ribs if there is a problem with brittle bones, but direct the breath towards the hands.

Cross the arms in front of the body, placing the hands over the lower rib cage each side, and breathe in deeply. Hold the breath and, without putting any pressure into the head, force the breath towards the hands while exerting some pressure on the sides of the rib cage.

Repeat several times. To ensure that filtrate from the lungs enters the lymph cistern, massage with the thumb from the edge of the rib cage in line with the nipple down towards the navel.

Do this exercise three times on each side.

If the above exercise proves difficult for young children and the elderly, the following alternative will be helpful:

Do-in gently up and down the rib cage, back and front (Fig. A2.3).

EXERCISE 3, INGUINAL DRAIN (Fig. A2.4)

This exercise clears the lymphatics of the small intestine, colon and the area around the rectum, as well as reducing any spasm that forms in the psoas muscles.

Roll up a medium-sized hand towel and place it in the right groin. Then, either sitting or lying, bend the right leg at the knee and pull it up towards the chest with both hands. Hold it there for about 10 seconds to allow the lymph to drain up into the lymph cistern.

(a)

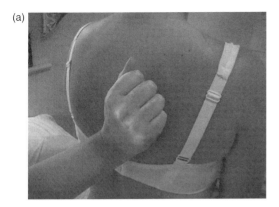

(b)

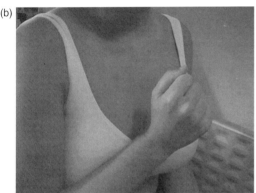

Figure A2.3 Alternative to Exercise 2: do-in to the rib cage (back and front).

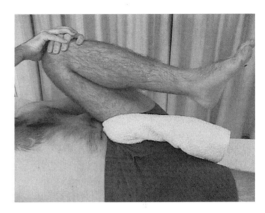

Figure A2.4 Exercise 3: inguinal drain.

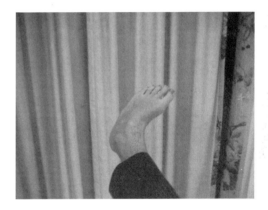

Figure A2.5 Foot rotations.

Then repeat the exercise with the left leg. This procedure should be repeated four more times.

FOOT ROTATION (Fig. A2.5)

This exercise stimulates the muscles of the thigh and activates the nerves restoring energy to the muscles and ligaments of the pelvis. This helps to release any compression of the sciatic nerve and, combined with Exercise 3, is very successful for pelvic and lower back conditions.

1. Lie face up on a bed with the right leg raised about 6 inches.
2. Rotate the raised foot at the ankle: ten times one way and ten times the other way.
3. Repeat with the left leg.

When this exercise is first performed, the rotating foot might shudder as it moves around, not quite forming a circle. However, as the nerve supplies in the pelvic region improve, so too will the ability to draw a perfect circle in the air with both feet. This outward sign signals the regeneration of interconnecting energy fields and repair. Ideally, this exercise should be carried out at home morning and evening. But, to a lesser degree, just rotating the ankles while sitting at a desk, at traffic lights or when watching the television will help enormously in keeping the energy fields vibrating.

Foot rotation and Exercise 3 (combined with reflexology, lymph drainage massage, Exercise 1 (lymph cistern) and do-in), would be beneficial before any long-haul flight. Foot rotation could then continue during the flight at half-hour intervals.

EXERCISE 4, THE FOUR-STEP EXERCISE (Fig. A2.6)

This exercise helps to stimulate the many nerve stations of the abdominal region and clear lymph nodes and vessels in the area.

1. **Step one:** with the tip of the right thumb at the base of the sternum, press the heel of the thumb down deep along the right edge of the rib cage. Exert abdominal pressure against the thumb several times for about 5 seconds. This forces the lymph into the lymph cistern, which must be cleared prior to further lymph drainage exercises.
2. **Step two:** exercise 1, lymph cistern.
3. **Step three:** repeat step one, but on the left edge of the rib cage.
4. **Step four:** repeat exercise 1, lymph cistern.

EXERCISE 5, THE BRONCHIAL PLEXUS (Fig. A2.7)

The bronchial plexus, which is on the artery supplying the bronchi and bronchiole, lies behind the sternum on the 3rd sternal groove. Stimulation of this plexus is achieved by clearing

(a)
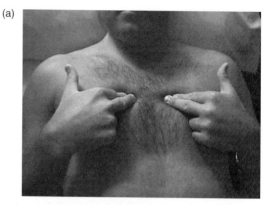

(b)
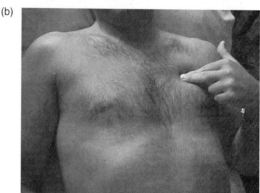

(c)
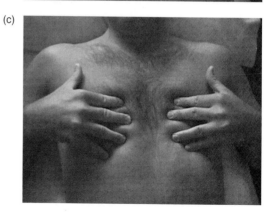

(a)
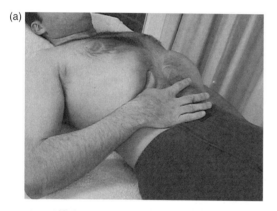

(b)
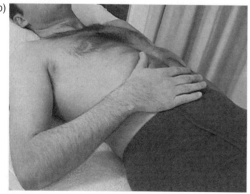

Figure A2.6 Exercise 4: the four-step exercise.

Figure A2.7 Exercise 5: the bronchial plexus.

the lymphatics behind the sternum using a simple massage:

1. Massage firmly with the fingertips along the third depression of the sternum for a few minutes. Then, moving down to the fourth depression, repeat the exercise to clear the bronchial lymph nodes.

2. Massage up along each side of the sternum, as this also helps to keep the parasternal lymph nodes clear too.

If you are using this massage technique as part of a maintenance program for asthma, it is very important not to repeat the exercise more than once during each treatment session. People with asthma should progress slowly and follow the treatment program in Chapter 12.

EXERCISE 6, THE BRAINSTEM
(Fig. A2.8)

This part of the brain acts as a highway for messages traveling between other parts of the brain and the spinal cord, but it also connects with 10 of the 12 pairs of cranial nerves and controls basic functions, such as breathing, vomiting and eye reflexes.

1. Insert the fingers or thumbs of both hands underneath the occipital bone at its center point and massage into the ridge (Fig. A2.8a).

2. Massage down the back of the neck to the 7th cervical vertebra, with its prominent spine (Fig. A2.8b,c), and return to the central starting point. Do this several times until you feel the muscles become supple under your fingers.

(a)
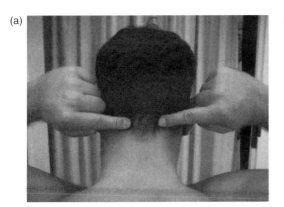

(b)
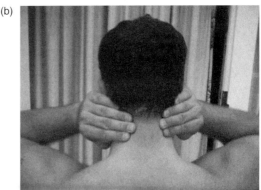

(c)
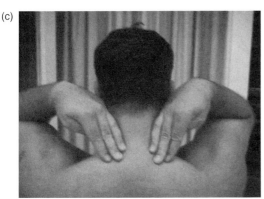

(d)
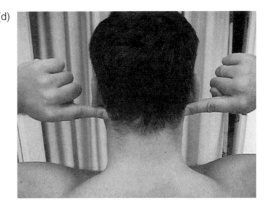

Figure A2.8 Exercise 6: the brainstem.

Return to the starting point and massage into the base of the skull, following the line until you reach the ears (Fig. A2.8d). Repeat a few times until these muscles too become supple. This massage appears to influence the energy fields of the vagus and phrenic nerves.

EXERCISE 7, LYMPH DRAINAGE OF THE HEART (Fig. A2.9)

Note: This exercise should be performed only after Exercises 2, 5 and 6, and never on its own.

The deepest lymph nodes lie just behind the 5th intercostal spaces (between the ribs) of the rib cage on each side of the sternum (breast bone) and out as far as below each nipple. The lymph from the left side drains under the sternum to the lymph nodes next to the sternum on the right. Lymph from the right side drains into the same area, and then, together, up through the lymphatics to the lymphatic duct behind the right clavicle.

Massage with the fingertips along the route of drainage. When this massage has been completed take a deep breath and hold it while you position the palm of your hand against the base of the breastbone. Press gently but firmly towards the heart, at the same time push the diaphragm out against the palm of your hand while holding the breath. You should feel pressure against your hand, hold this position for 6 seconds then relax. It is important that pressure is directed towards the hand and not the head. Repeat this exercise three more times. Eventually, you might hear a little gurgle in the small intestine or colon. This procedure is contraindicated in cardiac edema.

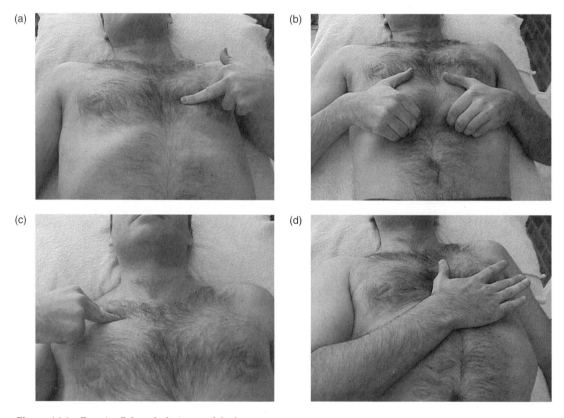

Figure A2.9 Exercise 7: lymph drainage of the heart.

EXERCISE 8, THE NERVE SUPPLY TO THE ISLETS OF LANGERHANS AND THE CARBOHYDRATE FUNCTION OF THE PANCREAS

Roll up a medium-sized hand towel, place it in the right groin, and then either sitting or lying, bend the right leg by the knee and pull it up towards the chest with both hands. Hold it there for about 10 seconds to allow the lymph to drain up into the lymph cistern. While in this position, push-out the abdomen against the towel and breathe in deeply. Repeat the exercise with the left leg. This procedure should be repeated four more times.

EXERCISE 9, THE DEEP INGUINAL NODES
(Fig. A2.10)

Exercises 8 and 9 can be of benefit where frequent urination is a problem and can enhance performance of the organs in the lower abdomen.

Press the heel of the right thumb or, if preferred, the side of the hand down into the hollow at the top of the right leg near the pubic bone. At the same time, draw-in the lower abdomen, as if to suck up the lymph from that area. Repeat three times. Then do the same with the left thumb on the left side.

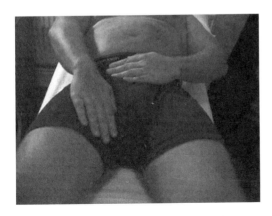

Figure A2.10 Exercise 9: the deep inguinal nodes.

EXERCISE 10, THYROID AND PARATHYROID LYMPH NODES
(Fig. A2.11)

1. Massage deep into the tissues above and below the clavicle several times, spending some time on the lymph drainage points (Fig. A2.11a).
2. Massage deep into the shoulder joint.

(a)

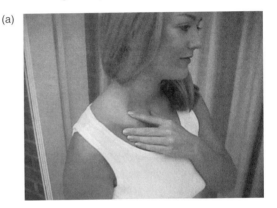

(b)

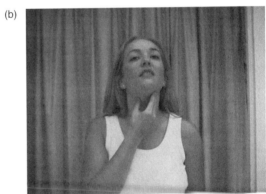

(c)

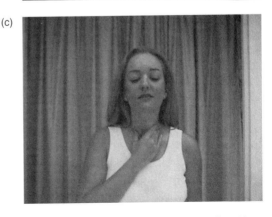

Figure A2.11 Exercise 10: the thyroid and parathyroid lymph nodes.

3. Perform the red light massage (Fig. A2.12).

4. Place the left hand over the throat, with the thumb and middle finger resting just under the base of the jaw. Massage down both sides of the larynx and out along the clavicle above and below. Do exactly the same with the other hand (Fig. A2.11b,c).

SELF-HELP ABDOMINAL MASSAGE TECHNIQUE

Abdominal massage given by a trained therapist is most beneficial, although the simplified version presented here is quite adequate when done correctly. It is not advisable for an untrained person to attempt a full abdominal massage on an elderly person because of the location of the aorta. There must also be an awareness of the possibility of osteoporosis while working around the rib cage.

Sit in a chair with the back supported:

1. Starting on the right side, close to the groin, use small, gentle, circular movements with the fingertips, if this is comfortable, up to the rib cage, across the front of the body and down the left side. Do this simple movement a few times and you will feel the muscles under the fingers start to soften.

2. Follow the line of the rib cage with the fingers, massaging gently the soft tissue just beneath. Do this several times, increasing the depth of the massage as the muscles relax; this will ease any spasm that has formed in the duodenum.

3. Taking the left hand, cross it over the abdomen and push the fingers into the appendix area (situated on the right side about 2 inches from the groin), holding the right hand over the left to exert a little pressure. Push the abdomen out against the fingers and hold for 5 seconds. Repeat on the left side.

4. Return to the rib cage and massage the soft tissue beneath.

5. Finish with small, circular movements, starting once more from the right side close to the groin, up to the rib cage, across the front of the body and down the left side. Spend a few minutes massaging the center of the abdomen then relax for 5 minutes.

See Fig. S2.2 for illustrations (p 34).

THE RED LIGHT MASSAGE
(Fig. A2.12)

This exercise clears the cervical lymph nodes and so permits the cervical ganglia to function to their optimum ability. It is so called because massaging the sides of the neck can easily be done when sitting at traffic lights. As the thyroid and parathyroid glands depend upon nerve impulses from the cervical ganglia, it would be most beneficial for this exercise to become a daily activity for the prevention of other conditions. For instance, hypothyroidism (which causes tiredness and can contribute to obesity), hyperthyroidism (which can lead to weight loss), and osteoarthritis and osteoporosis (which are caused by faulty calcium metabolism), can all benefit from this massage. As the heart and lungs can also benefit from the energetic interaction that is encouraged by this massage, it can pay dividends to be rigorous in its application. It will, however, take about 3 weeks for the nerve impulses from the ganglia to return to normal.

With the flat of the fingers of the right hand, press quite firmly from just beneath the left ear to the hollow at the base of the neck. This is easier if you turn the head slightly to the right and follow the line behind the sternocleidomastoid muscle. Do this massage 15 times, then change hands and repeat the procedure on the other side of the neck.

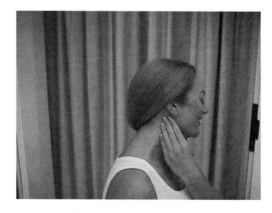

Figure A2.12 The red light massage.

GALL BLADDER EXERCISE

Note: Insulin-dependent diabetics should not use this technique.

This exercise can help enormously when reactive hypoglycemia is suspected.

Lean forwards and, with the fingertips of one or both hands, press up under the rib cage below the right breast to compress the gall bladder. Then push-out the abdomen against the fingertips once or twice.

This exercise can also help to correct any spasm in the abdominal muscles and intestines, thereby reinstating depleted energy to the muscles of the neck.

See Fig. 13.1, p 125 for an illustration of this technique.

THE ROWING BOAT EXERCISE
(Fig. A2.13)

This can be a bit difficult at first but is beneficial in helping to improve the nerve supply and tone to the muscles of the neck and upper spine.

1. Sit on a stool in front of a mirror with the back straight; imagine balancing a book on your head.

2. Hunch your shoulders so that your neck disappears and you can feel the base of the skull touching the top of the spine.

3. Bend the elbows and bring the arms, with clenched fists, level with the chest.

4. Slowly and deliberately push the elbows back, at the same time force the chest forwards and bring the head out from its sunken position, as though the head is being pulled upwards and the shoulders are about to touch each other behind the back.

5. Relax all the muscles by placing the hands, palm side up, on top of each other in the lap for a few seconds, breathing easily, before repeating the process.

This exercise should be repeated five times every morning and evening to encourage lymphatic drainage in the neck and shoulder region.

(a)
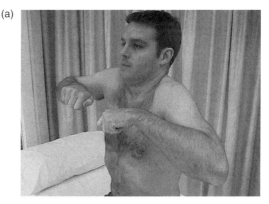

(b)
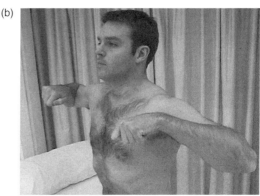

(c)
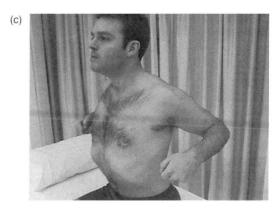

Figure A2.13 The rowing boat exercise.

STOMACH WASH

This exercise must always be preceded by reflexology to the liver, kidneys, spleen and lungs.

1. When the stomach is empty (preferably before getting out of bed in the morning) drink a glass of water, wait a few minutes and then lie on your back.

2. With the tips of the fingers, gently palpate under the sternum and to the left of the rib cage, until you hear the water gurgling.

3. Turn onto your right side for 3 minutes.

4. Turn back onto your back and palpate under the right side of the rib cage. Again, you might hear the water.

5. Turn onto your left side for 3 minutes.

6. Turn onto your back once more and palpate under the left side of the ribs down to the waist area. This also helps to clear the mesenteric plexus, which could help with constipation.

See Fig. 10.1a–c, p 82 for an illustration of this technique. This must not be carried out if the patient is experiencing reflux, the presence of blood in the stool, severe pain or under medical supervision without their doctor's advice.

THE SPLEEN, LIVER AND BILE SYSTEM ENERGIZER (Fig. A2.14)

Do-in works wonderfully here.

1. Tap the lower front of the rib cage with the fists loosely clenched or (if troubled with brittle bones) the flat of your hands from below the breasts to each side of the body five times.

2. Then, with the heel of the right hand, press-in the abdomen just below the right breast and push down a short distance towards the navel to clear the exit of the bile system.

THE SECRET OF BEAUTIFUL SKIN

1. **Red light massage:** do this massage 15 times, then change hands and repeat the procedure on the other side of the neck.

2. Place the index finger and thumb of both hands behind the ears so that each ear sits in the base of the index finger and middle finger.

3. Pull both hands firmly down the side of the face. Do this ten times.

(a)

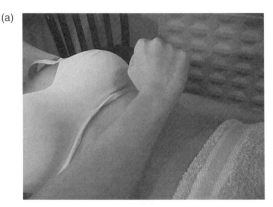

(b)

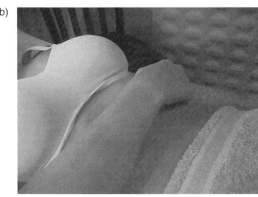

Figure A2.14 The spleen, liver and bile system energizer.

4. Place each thumb just below the ear and under the jawbone. Gently massage the space behind the jawbone, moving as you do towards the chin and finishing up with both thumbs just underneath the chin. Do this ten times.

5. Place each index finger either side of the bridge of the nose and massage in a circular motion down and under the cheekbones to the ears. *Note*: be careful about the amount of pressure you use in this area if you are prone to thread veins. Do this ten times.

6. Place each middle finger atop of the eyebrows and massage in a circular motion down towards each ear. Do this ten times.

7. With the pads of your fingers placed in the center of the forehead massage the center out and down towards the ears. Do this ten times.

8. Repeat step 2.

9. Repeat the red light massage and massage above and below the clavicles.

See Fig. 16.1 (pp 163–164) for an illustration of this technique.

Performing Exercise 6 after this face massage clears all of the lymph nodes that drain the scalp, face and external ear.

BREAST DRAIN

Follow the program on pp 50–52 and see Fig. 7.1.

1. **Exercise 1, lymph cistern.**
2. **The axillary nodes (armpits).**
3. **Breast drainage.**
4. **Reflexology.**

To help keep the axillary nodes clear on a daily basis: roll together a pair of gent's socks to form a ball and position the ball in the armpit. Press and hold the elbow firmly against the rib cage for 2–3 minutes.

THE BRAIN DRAIN

Follow the program as detailed on pp 149–151.

THYMUS (Fig. A2.15)

To clear the thymus, massage deeply behind the notch at the top of the sternum and across the first and second depressions as the lymph drains into the nodes on each side of the sternum. Massage into the drainage points.

DIAGNOSTIC TESTS

Note: The following tests are to be used as a guide. The patient is advised to consult their doctor if a problem is suspected.

Adrenal gland test (see p 165)

Thyroid test (see p 165)

Raised blood pressure

Practise this massage to the ring finger of the left hand. Enclose this finger between the thumb and

(a)

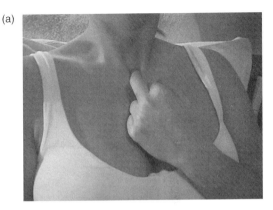

(b)

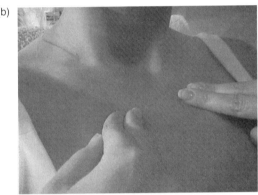

(c)

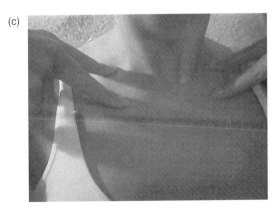

Figure A2.15 The thymus.

index finger of your right hand. From the second joint, massage downwards to the nail (see Fig. 13.2, p 127).

Exercise 6, the brainstem (Fig. A2.8, p 181) is also helpful.

List of suppliers

Aquamix
20 Orville Street, St Helens,
Merseyside WA9 3JJ
Tel: 01744 816990
Fax: 01744 816990
Suppliers of all types of water purification/filtration systems. Replacement membranes and cartridges for most makes.

Auro Organic Paints, Adhesives and Floor Care
Unit 1, Goldstones Farm, Ashdon,
Saffron Walden, Essex CB10 2LZ
Tel: 01799 584888
Fax: 01799 584042
Paints are made from natural materials, familiar to the human organism, which exclude additional irritants from modern chemistry. There is a full declaration of constituents on all Auro products. In addition, trial samples are available on request for customers to test for any individual intolerance. Mail order to anywhere in the UK.

Bio-Health Ltd
Culpeper Close, Medway City Estate, Rochester,
Kent ME2 4HU
Tel: 01634 290115
Fax: 01634 290761
Producers of vitamin, mineral and nutritional supplements that are totally free from chemical substances used as binders, fillers, excipients, flowing/caking agents, disintegrants, coloring, flavorings and preservatives. Supplements are manufactured to the highest standards using the purest ingredients and are suitable for adults and children and compatible with genuine holistic principles. The capsule contents quickly disperse, dissolving in the gastric juices, ensuring full utilization of the natural enzyme-assisted digestive process, giving total assimilation.

Delamere Dairy Goats Milk Products
Yew Tree Farm, Bexton Lane, Knutsford,
Cheshire WA16 9BH
Tel: 01565 632422
Fax: 01565 750468
Fresh pasteurized goats milk (full fat and semi-skimmed), yogurts, goats cream and butter.

eco-ball™
Birchwood House, Briar Lane, Croydon,
Surrey CR0 5AD
Tel: 0181 777 3121
Fax: 0181 777 3393
Hypoallergenic, antibacterial alternative to soap powder.

The Environmental Protection Agency (EPA)
Has developed the Healthy Home Test Kit, which measures even the smallest concentrations of formaldehyde. The kit is easy to use and comes with complete instructions. It can be obtained from ConnectiCOSH, 77 Huyshope Ave, Hartford,
CT 06106, USA.

Freshlands Health Store
198 Old Street, London EC1V 9FR
Tel: 0171 250 1708
Fax: 0171 490 3170
Suppliers of Clearspring organic macrobiotic quality miso.

General Dietary Ltd
PO Box 38, Kingston upon Thames,
Surrey KT2 7YP
Tel: 0181 336 2323
Fax: 0181 942 9274
ENER-G-RICE and ENER-G BROWN RICE and
maize bread, a wheat-free, dairy-free, gluten-free
alternative to wheat bread.

The Healthy House
Cold Harbour, Ruscombe, Stroud, Gloucestershire
GL6 6DA
Tel: 01453 752216
Fax: 01453 753533
Mail-order business specializing in products for
people with asthma, allergies, eczema and
environmental illness.

Hockeys
South Gorley, Fordingbridge, Hampshire SP6 2PW
Tel: 01425 652542
Fax: 01425 652662
Farm meats reared in natural environment.
Refrigerated delivery service into London, Essex,
Kent, etc.

Medivac Healthcare Ltd
Wilmslow House, Grove Way, Wilmslow,
Cheshire SK9 5AG
Tel: 01625 539401
Fax: 01625 539507
Protective barrier covers, vacuum cleaners,
dehumidifiers and other anti-dust-mite aids.

Patent Filtration Ltd
Unit G1, Chiltern Trading Estate, Grovebury Road,
Leighton Buzzard, Bedfordshire LU7 8TU
Tel: 01525 384858
Fax: 01525 370443
Producers of equipment capable of removing harmful
airborne pollutants and contaminants that aggravate
the causes of breathing difficulties.

Schmidt Natural Clothing
21 Post Horn Close, Forest Row,
East Sussex RH18 5DE
Tel: 01342 822169
Fax: 01342 822169
A wide range of mail-order undergarments and
sleepwear for adults, children and babies (nappies).
Children's eczema sleepsuits, certified organic cotton,
natural silk, finest merino. No bleaching agents, no
formaldehyde, no harmful dyes.

Simply Water Ltd
Environment House, Brighton Green,
Dublin 6, Eire
Tel: 01 4920414
Fax: 01 4920712
E-mail: info@simplywater.com
Fluoride reduction filter.

Sussex High Weald Dairy Products
Putlands Farm, Duddleswell, Uckfield,
East Sussex TN22 3BJ
Tel: 01825 712647
Fax: 01825 712474
Mail-order sheeps milk dairy products.

Vitacare Ltd
The Business Centre, 758–760 Great Cambridge
Road, Enfield, Middlesex EN1 3PN
Tel: 0181 443 7089
Fax: 0181 366 5576
'Nanny' goat milk infant nutrition.

Weleda (UK) Ltd
Heanor Road, Ilkeston, Derbyshire DE7 8DR
Tel: 0115 9448222
Fax: 0115 9448210
Suppliers of natural essential oils, homeopathic
remedies and natural toiletries. All products are free
from synthetic fragrances, colors and artificial
preservatives.

Index

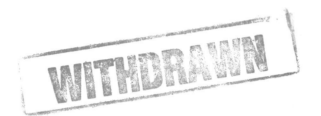

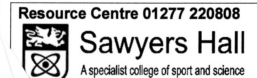